WHEN CALORIES

&

CARDIO DON'T CUT IT

JOANNE LEE CORNISH

Editor Stewart Hennessey

Printed in the United States of America

First Edition, 2018

ISBN 978 0 692 11273 1 (print)

978 0 692 11277 9 (ebook)

1482 N Foresto Bello Way

EAGLE

Idaho 83616

www.TheShrinkShop.com

www.JoanneLeeCornish.com 10 9 8 7 6 5 4 3 2 2

Dedicated to my husband

Kevin Cornish

I pinch myself every day

Until my last breath and beyond

ABOUT THIS BOOK

Losing weight is one of the greatest challenges a person may face in their lifetime. A thickening waistline that defies our best efforts affects our self confidence and we have no idea what to tell our kids so that they can avoid the same frustration.

We live in exciting times as we are now clear about what causes the physical changes we abhor and although calories and exercise play a role, they are deep in the shadows of the hugely dominant players who ultimately control what we weigh and what shape we take.

In "When Calories & Cardio Don't Cut It" you will learn

The one reaction that needs to occur for fat breakdown.

1. What causes fat storage to be accelerated by age.

2. The three times of life you can increase your number of fat cells.

3. Why Chronic dieters end up with fat arms and thick waists.

4. How to avoid weight gain in menopause (or man opause).

5. Why some fat is resistant to exercise

6. What triggers water retention and how to lose it overnight.

7. Why puberty is critical to the fat cell.

"When Calories & Cardio Don't Cut it" is a fascinating look at the major influencers that impact body composition and fat patterning. It explains how these players pay little heed to our obsessive tracking of intake vs expenditure and it will show you how you can control them to work in your favor.

Before you hang your hat on the next diet or go back to the one that 'worked before' take this opportunity to explore how to live lean for a lifetime. It is entirely possible and extremely probable with the right know how.

CONTENTS

PREFACE

I have been writing diets for decades. Back before the apps and programs, it was just me a pencil, some paper and my trusted calculator.

The diets were good, and people got great results. So why did the same people keep coming back for a new diet?

Losing weight can be the biggest challenge of one's life. It's not particularly fun, and it can take a long time. I was giving my clients a great product, but their success hinged on their motivation to stick to the plan. Research confirms that willpower, on average, lasts about three weeks. Like a muscle it gets tired, worn out and exhausted.

I have always enjoyed reading about nutrition and how the body works. It is a little like a jigsaw puzzle to me, putting the pieces together till a real picture transpires. Although it fascinated me, I hadn't thought that maybe my clients might be interested as well.

In 2005 I started to put together a seminar series called "If Diets Worked We'd All Be Skinny." Over five presentations I covered everything from childhood obesity to water retention, stress, lack of sleep, digestion and why most diets do not work.

I promoted the first presentation the best I knew how and presented to a handful of friends who were kind enough to turn up and support me. The second presentation there were a few unfamiliar faces, and by the time I did the fifth seminar there wasn't standing room. Then I was asked to repeat the whole series, which I did to a full house every time.

Maybe people were as fascinated as I was about the ins and outs of body composition, aging and nutrition. That year I restructured my business; instead of just giving out great diets, I took the time to explain the diets. We have known for a long time how and why the body stores fat, and we have known for many decades the process of fat breakdown, but nobody at that time seemed to be talking about it.

Like me, maybe other coaches just assumed their clients had no interest? Or maybe it was too much like hard work, as it took a greater investment of energy and time on my part.

Clients would leave our first meeting excited, they would send friends to meet with me, they sent their kids, they sent their bosses to see me. I was designing diets very similar to the ones I had given out in the past, but now I had long term compliance. I had many people come and see me and I would never see them again. Later I would get an email thanking me and telling me how much weight they had lost.

Perhaps that's why other coaches don't take this approach as it's not the best way to hold onto a client. The weight loss industry is a huge and very profitable business with an enormous failure rate. It is an industry that succeeds on repeat business because when the diet fails, the consumer blames themselves and not the product.

I don't want to heap scorn on the weight loss industry as there are some really good programs out there but, like my diets back in the day, most fail to provide the client with the understanding they need to get them through the long haul that lies ahead of them.

My epiphany was that if you give a person good, valid information that they can relate to, then they will make better decisions all by themselves. Hence this book was born.

Fast forward, and I have written the content for this book, so it was time to find an editor. I was referred (thank you Mark) to an English based website called peopleperhour.com, I submitted my project and whittled the responses down to four editors. I sent each a different chapter thinking that I would see which one I liked the best and would go from there. One guy criticized just about everything I sent him, which was a little disheartening. One lady asked that even if I didn't choose her could I please send her more chapters as it was so interesting. Editor number three asked if she could send their chapter to a nephew who could really use the information. Now I was feeling a lot better about myself, but it was editor number four that stole my heart. Stewart Hennessey lives in Scotland, a very well established editor who showed a lot of patience with a newbie writer like me. Stewart lost a stone (14lb) while editing this book, not once did I "tell" him what to do; he just took the information and ran with it.

And that is what I hope this book does for you. You won't find any meal plans in this book; you won't find food exchanges or report cards to fill in. What you will find is the information you need to implement the changes necessary to make a permanent shift in your body composition and overall health. What you will find in this book is knowledge you can share with your family, your parents, your friends and your kids.

I am told that I have a way of taking complicated information and making it relatable. I simplify some very complex processes, and I know some scholars out there will criticize me for it. I would counter that this is part of the problem. We are either given no information at all, or the information available is so long winded, complex, confusing and even contradictory that it is not helpful. I hope I have found a middle ground.

Bottom line: I have worked with people one on one for decades. I have worked with every personality type you can imagine, and I believe I have found a way to communicate what is needed in a fun, fascinating and intriguing way.

We only take so many breathes in this life, and I hope the time you spend reading my work is time well spent; that would make me very happy :)

Joanne

HOW TO READ THIS BOOK

To make this book a little easier to navigate I have used text boxes.

Text within a box represents what is useful to understand. If some of my work gets too detailed for your taste, simply refer to the summaries in the text box. All the important points are there.

You will also see paragraphs in italics.

Text in italics contains information you might find interesting but is not essential for a general understanding. From time to time I will tackle a topic in depth. The detail may be a little too much for some readers, in which case pay it no heed; just skim over and keep going.

If by the end of the book you want to give me a pat on the back, shake my hand or give me a fist pump, please do, here's how:

Review me on Amazon (it's a big deal)

www.caloriesandcardio.com

www.joanneleecornishauthor.com

INTRODUCTION

Like most people, I am uneasy about animal experiments and utterly horrified by the idea of painful experiments on humans which, of course, are illegal throughout the modern world. However, during the dark days of World War Two when the world was in chaos, and famine stalked continents, the US authorities wanted to understand the effects of starvation.

A brutal experiment was conducted, from 19 November 1944 to 20 December 1945, in which 36 men were "starved" for months and observed carefully throughout. The results of this experiment – which can never be repeated – speak volumes about human behavior, our bodies and our relationship with food.

The men were all conscientious objectors who volunteered for the experiment which was carried out in Minnesota. (Even at the time, what became known as the Minnesota semi starvation study was thought by many to be unethical.) The full results were only made public in 1950, it a two volume tome consisting of 1,385 pages.

However, hard facts were well known by 1946 when the US was already helping millions around the world recover from starvation. In essence, the results contradict all the baloney about diets that has been forced on an unsuspecting public during the decades since that global upheaval.

Although the Minnesota semi starvation study was intended for a grand and meaningful purpose, it is instructive in today's world, at least to anyone who has struggled not just with involuntary starvation but with the pressure to attain a certain physical look.

The Minnesota study was not about showing that starvation is bad for you – everyone, from the cavemen on, knew that – but about precisely how we relate to food, both mentally and physically. For anyone who has ever been on a diet or been around somebody on a diet, I believe much of the following will hit home.

We all know that we cannot fully rely on studies, especially studies over 70 years old, yet this is that rarity; research which stands the test of time.

In the Minnesota study, run by Prof. Ancel Keyes, the 36 men of healthy mind and body spent the first three months eating normally, while their behavior, personality and eating patterns were noted in great detail. This was followed by six months during which the men were restricted to approximately half of their daily intake, which was about 1500 calories (a pretty conservative intake by today's standards). During the six months, the men lost about 25% of their body weight.

This was followed by three months of revocation, during which various rehabilitative diets were tried to re nourish the volunteers. Several the volunteers continued to be studied for almost nine months following the six months of restrictions.

The men experienced dramatic changes which, in many cases, lasted well into the rehabilitation phase. (When contemplating this, it might be instructive to consider your own behavior and the behavior of others while on a diet, bearing in mind that these were healthy men without a history of restriction. We can shudder while thinking of the cumulative effects on those who do one diet after another.)

There was a dramatic increase in the men's interest in food. They thought about food continually and dreamt about food. They talked non stop about food. They read about food. They collected cookbooks and stared at photographs of food. This increased interest correlated with a decline in interest in all other activities and aspects of life.

The men toyed with the food they smuggled out of the dining room to eat alone when, in long, drawn out rituals, they would make meals last two hours; these were meals that should have taken minutes. They studied food production processes, and they researched menus. They grew interested in nutrition and even in agriculture. They gained pleasure from watching other people eat, and some of the men began collecting food paraphernalia like kitchen utensils and plates. They started by hoarding these items, and then they just began hoarding in general; this included purchases that were completely meaningless. Following the study, this behavior totally puzzled the men involved.

When asked about what they would do after the experiment 40% of the men said that cooking was one of their future plans. Interestingly, after the study, a few of the men did indeed become chefs or went on to work in agriculture.

They started to drink a lot of coffee and tea, which got out of hand and had to be limited to nine cups a day. Chewing gum also got out of hand, with one man chewing through 40 packs a day.

Not surprisingly, all of the men experienced hunger. Some did okay with this, and yet some experienced a total loss of control. Many of the men binged. One man working in a grocery store completely lost it and binged on cookies and popcorn and developed severe self loathing. Another man had to leave the study as he would eat an enormous amount of food, become sick, go back to eating an enormous amount of food, become sick and just go through the cycle endlessly.

Most of the men could not control their appetite. During the three months of rehabilitation, many basically ate continuously. Even after the three months of refeeding some men still felt hungry after a meal. The refeeding phase was not paltry; it was not uncommon for the men to be eating 8,000 to 10,000 calories a day.

What became clear from all this is the regulatory systems – which have since been more fully discovered and defined – that govern hunger and fullness were thrown into disarray by the six months of restriction. Steady eating habits keep the body and mind happy. Punishing diets are just maddening, albeit less maddening if they are less punishing; but the regulatory systems are still going doolally to some extent.

Men would eat until they were bursting. Some had to separate themselves from food altogether as they felt they had no control whatsoever. Those who had happily eaten three meals a day now ate six. And some ate until they could no longer swallow.

It took more than eight months after the refeeding phase of the study for most of the men to return to normal eating patterns. Remember: the 36 men were selected because they were both physically and psychologically healthy.

Most experienced great emotional distress during the study. At least 20% of the men suffered such emotional distress that they were not able to function properly. Many suffered extreme depression, some experienced extreme mood swings with extreme highs and extreme lows. Symptoms included irritability, anger, negativity, argumentativeness, nail biting, smoking and neglect when it came to personal hygiene.

After two weeks of refeeding, this is one man's report: "I have been more depressed than ever in my life.... I thought that there was only one thing that would pull me out of the doldrums, that is release from C.P.S. [the experiment] I decided to get rid of some fingers. Ten days ago, I jacked up my car and let the car fall on these fingers.... It was premeditated."

This man did indeed cut off three of his fingers. Another man suffered such extreme personality disturbances that he had to leave the study in week ten. And he had only lost ten pounds of his original body weight.

The men became withdrawn and isolated. They lost their sense of humor. They lost the sense of friendship with each other and felt increasingly inadequate. They became less interested in women and those with relationships found them very strained. One man reported it was just too much trouble to see his girlfriend. And if they went to see a show the most interesting part for him was always when there were scenes of people eating.

The men's interest in sex plummeted, with one man stating he had "no more sexual feeling than a sick oyster". You might think that this interest would be the first to return after the experiment, yet even after three months, the men judged themselves to be far from normal in this area.

The men reported difficulty in concentrating, in alertness and comprehension. They experienced intestinal discomfort, less need for sleep, headaches, and sensitivity to noise and light. They reported the loss of physical strength as well as bloating and water retention, hair loss, vision problems and intolerance to cold temperatures.

BMR stands for basal metabolic rate, and this is the amount of energy calories the body needs at rest. We want our BMR to be high as this means we are using a lot of energy. In the Minnesota semi starvation study, the men's BMR's dropped by about 40%, showing their bodies had adapted to the restricted calories. Interestingly, during the refeeding phase those men who gradually increased their calorific intake had no BMR increase for three weeks, whereas those men who ate large amounts of food asap increased their metabolic rate.

I am sure that some readers can relate very personally to (hopefully much less extreme!) versions of what these men experienced. Having spent 13 years of my life competing, and dieting for maybe half of that time, I can certainly relate to it. As I scroll through social media how many times do I see a photograph of somebody's meal? As a trainer, how many clients have brought me food that they would never eat themselves? As we restrict our food, our fascination with it increases and can become obsessional.

I watch fitness competitors isolate themselves before an upcoming show, unable to deal with anything other than meal prep and the next workout. I see many of them desperately unhappy; I see how they became intolerant to certain foods and used the word "bloat" many times in every conversation.

Post diet, many suffer a massive rebound in weight which does not help with their depressed state. The real sadness is that this is expected and accepted, and before the body has even had the chance to recover they embark on the next diet.

The Minnesota semi starvation study was 36 healthy men without a history of food restriction. It is a study that is very unlikely ever to be repeated. We can only surmise about what occurs with years or decades of repeated dieting.

The body and the mind have an incredible capacity to adapt to energy deprivation, and when we lose weight the body doesn't automatically stay at this low weight. Regulatory systems have a bias for weight gain and, as the study shows, the mind and body work against rapid weight loss.

To conclude the men's journey: following the experiment, the men regained the weight they had lost plus, on average, another 10%. Over the following six months they slowly returned to their original body weight.

I include this study here partly just because I believe it is a bold illumination of commonplace patterns and I hope it frees some of you from feelings of inadequacy and self blame. Upliftingly, the Minnesota study does not suggest for one minute that weight loss is impossible or even particularly difficult. It simply reveals that we must work with our body, not against it. In relation to this I coined a phrase during a seminar series I wrote many years ago, and I still believe it sums up our silly battles with our bodies; "The body is way smarter than our dumb actions."

And as we know, all of us can be rather dumb at times. For many people, if they had three wishes then the perfect healthy body would very likely be one of those three. Despite this heartfelt desire, the majority of people come nowhere near close to hitting the mark.

This is not merely a dumb contradiction between desire and achievement. It is also simple ignorance, which is hardly surprising since we are never taught any low key truths about our physical and mental well being's intimate relationship with food. We are bombarded all our lives by marketing hyperbole; media scare stories and confusing and conflicting theories which are invariably overstated. It's little wonder we are clueless when it comes to the plain truth about food intake. Nobody has ever taught us.

At my nutrition business in Santa Monica, California I have sat across the table from all sorts of people who I might once have found very intimidating; doctors, university professors, a great many athletes, MBAs, PhDs, celebs, millionaires and even billionaires; the common denominator has been that none have ever been taught squat about nutrition. These hugely successful people ask the same sort of naive questions that regular folk might ask.

There was the 35 year old bride to be, a successful established professional lady who worked out ferociously; she looked quite trim and told me from the get go that she followed a very low carbohydrate diet and she wanted help fine tuning that diet for her wedding day. Thinking that she had a good grip on nutrition I started my spiel a little farther in than I would normally start. After about 25 minutes, she made it plain that she firmly believed cheese was a carbohydrate. I stopped dead in my verbal tracks; she was following a low carb diet and did not know that cheese was not a carb? It turned out that she thought carbs were bread and only bread; she was on a no bread diet. (It was pretty cool for me; given somebody that disciplined with a wedding day fast approaching, I was able to turn the tide with ease, such that she dropped two sizes before the big day.)

There was also a 16 year old student who came to see me and straight up said she had no clue how to eat. She was also a very smart young lady, but she told me she was constantly tired during the day and had no idea how to make good food choices. She wanted to be more prepared for when she went to college in a few years. Being 30 years her senior, and not having teenagers of my own to ask, I was curious if even basic nutrition was part of her education. It was not and never had been. She knew precisely nothing about it.

There was a cardiologist who told me he had received a one hour class on nutrition; no more, in all his years at medical school. He was fun to work with as I was able to pick his brains. We made two simple changes, and he dropped 14 pounds in the first month.

I'm conveying these vignettes to show you that you are not alone if you feel confused, ill informed or even ignorant. The good news is that with the simple and correct information about body composition and health, all of these people could make lifelong changes to their bodies and eating behavior. There was no need for mad fad diets or starvation or tasteless concoctions or anything at all abnormal. It was just about becoming informed. I continually shoot my nutrition business in the foot by basing my success on clients no longer needing me.

With the majority of people, noncompliance is a perfectly natural result of not understanding, and therefore not believing in what you've been instructed to do. In other words, if you don't understand what you are doing you are unlikely to get it done, and this most certainly applies to weight loss. I find this is most common with intelligent people. You cannot just tell somebody with an active, sharp, curious mind what to do and expect them just to do it unendingly and unquestioningly. It is vital to give intelligent people good information if you are asking them to implement long term changes to their bodies, behavior, and lives.

It's a little like giving a man a fish so he won't be hungry but teach a man to fish and he'll never be hungry again.

As I say, we are not taught about nutrition, and even the most preoccupied class member would grasp a few helpful basics if we were. I could vent and rant for pages about this missed opportunity. It needn't be a matter of boring schoolchildren to tears with endless hours of detailed study; just some basic information on nutrition, body composition and health. The more biologically inclined could pursue it further if the class piqued their interest. It would put me out of business, so maybe I should be mercenary and grateful for the uniformed innocents who file through my door. But it makes me sad that young people of today are not being taught how to eat healthily, all the while they are being bombarded with manipulating marketing, quick fix products and new daft fads and theories that promise them that photoshopped body they envy on Instagram.

In this book, I would like to provide you with the information you need to make a permanent shift in your health and body composition. I cannot promise you the physique you asked for with one of your three wishes. Just as I cannot turn a blonde into a brunette, I cannot turn one body type into another. But I can explain it, and help you get the best out of your body.

I aim to simplify some pretty complex information. The experts and researchers know a lot, but they can leave their readers behind with unnecessary detail and in depth biology. I am here for every person who wants a great body and tip top health, the person who is willing to do the work and who is fed up being bamboozled by all the media hysteria, marketing overstatement, and contradictory nonsense.

CHAPTER ONE: FOODY BUSINESS

Health and food is a subject that has been written into the ground, but please bear with me here. We need to touch base with the basics of food because the food is itself the basis for healthy living – and unhealthy living. The difference between healthy and unhealthy living involves choices which are not nearly as tough as neurotic fanatics might have you believe.

That's not the only good news. Fact is: we have reached a point where food and health have been thoroughly and properly researched. We know a lot of facts for certain. My humble contributions to the field are based on decades of observation, and although I will be squaring my experience with hard scientific research, I would emphasize that what I am doing here is distilling research. I will be drawing on the work of scientists who write lengthy papers, so you don't have to wade through them all.

When it comes to food – the lovely stuff of life – we must peer through the alarmist media fog. We must ignore all the hysterical overstatements, scare stories, fad diets, miracle solutions and associated nonsenses which serve to make us all anxious. Then a clear picture emerges. We need not feel overwhelmed. We easily know enough to make wise choices regarding longevity, easy weight loss, physical strength and general well being, and we can make these choices without confining ourselves to an unsustainably puritan diet or fretting about every calorie that crosses our lips.

So, in this opening chapter, I offer the fruits of good scientific research, and with all respect and thanks to the men and women who devoted their time and minds to proper research. It is unfortunate that over the years much good work has got hijacked, misrepresented and spun for dramatic effect.

I have worked in the health industry all my adult life. I think it is a fun challenge and a potentially fascinating subject; not a matter of worry, defeatism and mind numbing lectures. I have watched people's bodies balloon and shrink, go from poor health to excellent health, and vice versa, and I have watched bodies weather the ravages of age, sometimes lamentably, sometimes with grace. There is absolutely no doubt that having a body which looks and feels good, and which works magnificently, is a simple matter of lifestyle choices.

Sadly, we are confused and overloaded with information, much of which is dubious. The excessive amount of conflicting information often leads to nonaction, so if you want a healthy body – the happy bedfellow of a healthy mind – then some fundamental facts about food are essential. We'll get to more fun lifestyle stuff afterward.

The truth is I shouldn't have to write this food chapter at all. At some point in our education, we should all have been taught this – it's not rocket science. Had we all been taught about food, nutrition and health, we would avoid so much of the frustration and confusion we only get around to facing when we are adults.

At the risk of sounding evangelical, it is true to say that if people were taught to understand food at an early age, there would be an effortless and natural shift towards good health, in just one generation. Moreover, growing up and becoming body conscious would be a lot less arduous if children and teenagers were not prey to the weight loss, fitness and food industries. Melodrama, fake photos and the dodgy use of stats create a stress that should not be loaded onto our youth.

Fear, hope, anger, and excitement are all deployed to shift products off shelves, and honest perspective is lucky to get a look in. I hope in the following chapters to provide you with information that is valid, stands up to scrutiny and which you can relate to.

So, necessity demands that I start with the basics about food: the foundation needed to get the most from this book.

So – you at the back! – pay attention, and let class commence.

SECTION 1: FOOD, THE STUFF OF LIFE

Most people struggle with their health and body requirements because they don't relate food to the quality of their life. Although we know it, and are often reminded of it, somehow, it's difficult to comprehend how the food we swallow can change our mood, create energy, reduce pain, feed disease and create unsightly rolls.

Naturally, understanding comes before belief, and therefore many people cannot truly believe what is possible through food, simply because they don't understand food.

The confusion is exacerbated when we are bamboozled – deliberately at times – by the expectation that we should know a lot about food. We read articles about eating more "whole grains", reducing "saturated fat" or "increasing protein" and yet no purveyor of foods takes the time to explain exactly what these apparently vital things are. We feel embarrassed asking about terms which are seemingly understood by all and sundry. The language of food and health was never taught to us during our formal education in high school, so why would we be familiar with it?

I had a nutrition client, an incredibly successful gentleman, who has asked me if an egg was a carbohydrate. Come to think, he is just one of many intelligent people who has asked me tragically ill informed questions. I have long ago learned to keep my jaw from dropping. The trouble is that people can come to believe nonsense that is much harder to put right because the factual error lies in that realm beyond simple food categories.

When people find a way of eating that works for them it can become very personal, a belief that they hold at their very core. Beliefs are very hard to change as they are central to an individual's self image. Alternative information that conflicts with a belief is shunned and ignored without investigation.

A coach or mentor can become so passionate about their beliefs that they force them on others. It may be a plant based diet, a gluten free diet, food combining, low glycemic, Paleolithic, grapefruit cabbage… and so on forever. What I would ask you to understand is that food and eating is a very emotional topic; people can be very aggressive in pushing their bias.

People are not unique. Human physiology and the way we handle our food is well understood nowadays. There is no "tricking" the body or dodging a hormone. There is a consequence for every action and the body – a thing of wonder – has an arsenal of weaponry to counteract some of the stupid things we do in the quest for a beach ready body.

Let's start with an explanation of what types of food there are, where they go when swallowed, what effect they have and where they end up.

MACRONUTRIENTS

Macronutrients are the nutrients we need in large amounts; for energy, growth and other bodily functions. The three macronutrients are:

PROTEIN (amino acids)

FAT (lipids)

CARBOHYDRATES (sugar)

Every food that we eat is designated one of these three macronutrients. Most naturally occurring foods contain more than one macronutrient, yet they will be described by the most dominant one.

A piece of beef is classed as a protein, but it also contains fat. Rice is known as a carbohydrate, yet it also contains protein. This is one of the ways people get confused. They read the labels and see that their peanut butter contains protein, so does their oatmeal and their bread, so how are you supposed to know that peanut butter is a fat and the cereals, and the bread are most definitely carbohydrates?

PROTEIN, THE GOOD, THE BAD AND THE GROSS

What is protein? If it HAD a face, took a breath and made a noise it is a protein. If it CAME from something that had a face, took a breath and made a noise, it is a protein. (Apologies if this sounds gross but the direct approach is often the most memorable.) So, it could be the chicken or the egg, it could be the cow or the milk.

There are most certainly plant based proteins but to state a simple fact: if it is an animal or came from an animal, it's protein.

COMPLETE V INCOMPLETE PROTEIN

Food cannot be used by the body in the form it takes on our plate. A piece of chicken does not enter our blood as a piece of chicken. When we eat that piece of chicken, we break it down (digest) into small single parts that are able to travel in the blood. Protein is broken down into amino acids (AA).

Be clear about this concept. When we put water in the freezer, it becomes ice. Water and ice; two words for the same thing in a different form. We eat protein; it is digested and enters our blood as amino acids.

Some amino acids are nonessential because the body can make them. However, there are nine amino acids which are essential amino acids (EAA), because the body cannot make them. They must come from food.

"Complete" proteins have all nine amino acids in them. There are other protein sources such as the protein we find in that peanut butter or the oatmeal or the bread or the vegetables, and these are incomplete proteins because they do not contain all of the essential amino acids.

Complete proteins that have all nine EAAs are superior to incomplete proteins (I know there are some vegans jumping up and down right now, but please hold your horses, I will expand on this... Did I mention food bias can be incredibly emotional?)

For the protein to be effectively used by the body it is preferred that all essential amino acids are present; it is for this reason that complete proteins are superior. All animal proteins are complete proteins, whether it is the animal itself or something the animal produces (milk, eggs). Plant based complete proteins include soy, quinoa, hemp, chia, and buckwheat.

Red meat contains heme iron. Heme iron is better absorbed than the non heme iron found in plants.

Animal protein also contains riboflavin, niacin, B6, B12, zinc and selenium.

It would be a challenge to find such an array of vitamins and minerals in processed meats. So many people get the majority of their protein from hot dogs, sausage, bacon, deli meat, jerky, pre made burgers, etc.

There is a concern about protein intake and illness, including cancer. How we handle our meats is important, and over cooking can be problematic. The heat of cooking releases fat and when this fat drops onto a cooking surface it produces polycyclic aromatic hydrocarbons which then seep back into the meat. PAHs have recognized carcinogens, but they are easily avoided by wiping up the fatty drips created during cooking. For those of you who like to grill, simply wipe underneath as you cook. If you like your meat very well done, then make sure you cut off those crusty bits. Heterocyclic amines are created when meat is cooked so well that crust is formed.

The link between animal protein and sickness seems to be associated with consuming processed proteins and eating over cooked meats. White meat has no such association, although how the animal was raised, and fed cannot be overlooked.

Processed meats (and processed food in general) are linked to inflammation, and inflammation is the underlying cause of many diseases, including heart disease and Alzheimer's. Inflammation is one way the body tries to protect itself from foreign substances, stress, infection, and toxic chemicals. When the immune system senses such dangers, the body activates proteins (yep proteins) to go and protect its cells.

Inflammation is a natural part of healing but, like anything, when it overreacts it can cause trouble. It can damage your gut, hurt your joints, damage blood vessels and cause autoimmune diseases. It will mess with your sleep, make weight loss a real issue and increase your chances of getting cancer.

Overeating processed foods will overload your body with substances it does not recognize, and this will put the immune system into overdrive. A large part of the connection between protein intake and sickness is the inclusion of processed meats in the studies.

NO MEAT, NO PROBLEM

Most vegans I have met are very well informed when it comes to food. They are confident about their food choices because they are educated about their food choices. I have to admire any group of people who live their lives based on their beliefs and not merely on their desires. When they look at the incomplete proteins, meaning those that are missing one or more of the essential amino acids, they know which incomplete proteins they can combine with other incomplete proteins to provide all essential amino acids at the same time. There are web pages dedicated to these combinations. Two of the best known combinations are rice and beans, and peanut butter and bread. When two incomplete proteins are combined, they can provide all the essential amino acids for the body to use.

Vegans are nearly always knowledgeable about their food, but the same cannot be said of vegetarians. I totally understand the repulsion to eat an animal. I often find myself on the cusp of vegetarianism and I know many other meat eaters who feel the same way. Then, in my nutrition practice, I meet those who chose to be vegetarian to lose weight. Weight loss is more challenging for vegetarians. It is certainly not impossible but replacing protein with carbohydrates, as many vegetarians do, moves you away from your goal, not closer to it. (All will be explained in the chapters to follow.)

It is important to remember that when you see 'protein' on a label, not all proteins are equal. The type and quality of a protein may be of paramount importance to attaining your goal. If you want to build muscle, it is best to eat high quality complete animal proteins, and if you want to avoid eating animal products, then it would be best to eat a wide variety of plant based complete and incomplete proteins.

WHAT DOES PROTEIN DO?

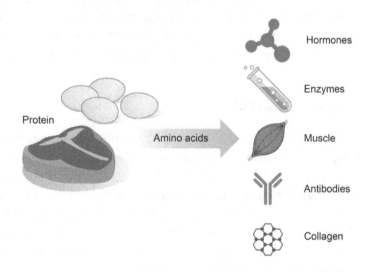

The protein that we eat is used to make enzymes (enzymes help make reactions in the body happen), antibodies, hormones, muscle, and collagen. The process we mostly associate with protein is, of course, building muscle. Protein plays a much larger role in our health and well being.

Protein cannot be absorbed and used by our body in its dietary state. We don't have chicken, eggs or even tofu floating around in our blood; we have amino acids. Amino acids make up every cell in our body.

We cannot store protein. As soon as we eat protein, it is broken down/digested, absorbed and utilized to make the enzymes, hormones, muscle, etc.

All proteins are made up of the nonessential and/or essential amino acids, and different proteins have different ratios of each of these amino acids. Problems can arise from eating the same foods over and over. An ultra narrow diet means getting the same amino acid profile every time. There is a benefit to eating a variety of different proteins to avoid a deficiency of any one amino acid.

Nitrogen is needed by every cell in our bodies, and we get nitrogen from the protein we eat. The more nitrogen there is in protein, the better the protein. We know we have complete and incomplete proteins, and proteins can then be ranked by the amount of nitrogen they provide. Soy is indeed a complete protein, but it is inferior to nitrogen rich milk, eggs, meat, and poultry. If building muscle is your goal, you should consider increasing your consumption of nitrogen rich complete proteins. The most nitrogen rich proteins include meat, fish, eggs, and milk.

Protein is our maintenance man, constantly building, maintaining and repairing. At the same time as protein is being used to build, protein is also being broken down by different processes in our body. "Nitrogen Balance" is where we have as much nitrogen entering our body as is being broken down.

Again, for muscle building, you want to make sure you have a "positive nitrogen balance," with more protein entering the body than is being broken down.

Because protein is always being used and never stored, I would suggest trying to eat protein several times a day. This is how protein differs from carbohydrates and fat, both of which can be stored (more on that later...).

You are what you eat, and this goes for animals too. If an animal has been pumped full of drugs and fed crap, then you might want to consider that before you eat that animal. Animals are kept in heinous conditions and fed food they were never meant to eat. They are sick, full of antibiotics and highly stressed, and then we eat their flesh or drink the milk. Hopefully one day soon, it will be realized and regulated as the highly unethical and potentially dangerous sourcing of food that it is.

There is a strong and welcome surge, pushing for ethically kept and healthfully fed animals. Unfortunately, these price point still tends to dictate conditions for animals, but things are improving, and if the push continues we might find quality protein produce readily available to everyone at reasonable prices.

This flows neatly into the critical issue of cost and our eating habits. Animals (including fish) had a face, took a breath, were born into life and thankfully this bestows value upon them. Protein is more expensive than any boxed or packaged product. To buy rice, pasta or bread is relatively inexpensive. When cost is a factor, it makes financial sense to buy less protein and more cereals, grains, etc. When we eat out we get a pasta dish with a little bit of protein thrown in, or that Chinese meal with mountains of rice and the shrimp you have to dig for.

Protein is expensive, and it makes sense for the restaurant business to focus their meals on the cheaper macronutrients. They skimp on the protein and rely heavily on the cheaper carbohydrates.

We have choices in the sourcing of our animal protein. The more we select the grass fed produce which is hormone, antibiotic and cage free, the more we empower the local and ethical farmer, and the more pressure we put on the monstrous giants of the food industry. Do not underestimate your power as a consumer. Collectively, people can really shake things up.

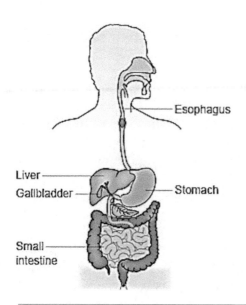

Liver
Gallbladder
Esophagus
Stomach
Small intestine

There is often a disconnect when people relate the food that they eat to their health, their energy, and their body composition. We like to throw around words like "metabolism" "body type" and "genetics" to explain our place in life. Most people don't know what any of those terms mean (why would they?), but they are still used as they remove any personal responsibility we might otherwise have.

To burst the bubble and shatter the matrix, metabolism, body type and genetics are all greatly influenced by the food that we eat. Ouch!... That was the weight of responsibility landing right back on your shoulders.

- Protein builds, maintains, repairs and creates. It is constantly required. It is being used and broken down all day and all night. It is the 24/7 maintenance man of your body.

- Protein is a source of nitrogen and every cell in our body needs nitrogen.

- There are complete and incomplete proteins, all of which are valuable although the complete proteins are better utilized.

- Protein cannot be stored. When we eat protein, it is used. There might be an advantage (depending on your goals) to eating protein several times a day.

- Protein is expensive, and usually, the least used macronutrient in a prepared meal.

- All complete proteins are not created equal. The level of nitrogen is ranked, and animal proteins rank higher than non-animal proteins.

To understand each macronutrient (protein, fat, carbohydrates) you need to know what happens to them once you have chewed them up and swallowed them. This is likely more than you need to know, but it completes the picture, removes question marks and joins the dots so to speak.

When it leaves your plate, protein is chewed and swallowed, moving down your esophagus (throat) and then entering your stomach. There it meets pepsin, an enzyme which breaks the protein and peptide bonds.

The majority of the digestion of protein happens in the small intestine. The pancreas is linked to the small intestine and sends pancreatic enzymes there to break down more peptide bonds (Trypsin, Chymotrypsin, Carboxypeptidase).

Polypeptides are broken down into peptides (two or more amino acids joined together) which are then broken down into single amino acids; a form in which they can then enter the bloodstream.

In a nutshell, protein is made up of many parts which the stomach and the small intestine break down into single units which can then enter the blood.

The single amino acids go straight to the liver. This organ takes what it needs before releasing the amino acids into the general bloodstream. Once in the general bloodstream, the amino acids can be used to make muscle, collagen, hormones, antibiotics and enzymes.

Complete digestion (breakdown) must take place for proteins to be fully utilized. When people have an issue digesting protein, they may be advised to take a supplement containing the enzyme pepsin.

We need a healthy stomach, pancreas, and liver for digestion to take place. Heavy use of antibiotics and over the counter pain medication can greatly affect the functionality of the stomach and liver.

FAT AND BIG FAT MISCONCEPTIONS

I first started competing in bodybuilding in the mid 1980s when fat was the devil. It was blamed for everything, from heart disease to saddle bags. Fat was the F word. Now, almost 40 years later we know how wrong we were. Fat is now fabulous, but it's going to take a long time to change the thinking that has been ingrained into us for decades. For many people, the calorie is still king, and because fat is more energy dense and has more calories per unit of weight than protein or carbohydrates, it still makes people nervous.

We can see it almost as a generational shift. My grandmother had no fear of fat, eating egg yolks, butter, full milk and plenty of fatty meat. My mother was brought up on these foods and yet as her generation grew up so did the food industry. Food became big business. Foods never seen on the table appeared thanks to improvements in transportation. My grandparents had the first television on their street, and within a few years they had multiple channels, and then along came the adverts; flogging food was now a big game.

Refrigeration, production, transportation and the microwave all brought new food choices to the family dining table. Women started to exercise, and the weight loss industry was born.

I started competing in the fitness world as a teenager and the best dieting advice I got from my mentor was to eat as little as possible and avoid fat completely.

My first competition diet at 18 years old was 800 calories a day and zero fat for the statutory 12 weeks.

I vividly remember, sitting in a chair at the gym, being told; "If you can eat less than that, even better."

I have no idea how I stuck to that diet, as I was also doing a business degree and working several nights a week. I put it down to having the energy of an 18 year old. I remember my grandmother being perplexed by the whole thing.

Today we know that fat is our fabulous friend, and my grandmother had been right all along with her whole eggs and cod liver oil, yet there is still resistance from my generation and the generation before me. Understandably, it is confusing as everything we were brought up with is being turned on its head. What they thought was right is now wrong and it's human nature to want to be right. Change is uncomfortable.

Jettisoning long held beliefs is difficult. People don't want the beliefs they were brought up with to be wrong. It would mean they had been making wrong choices all their lives, and no one wants that to be true.

You cannot be persuaded or bribed away from a belief. Beliefs lie at the very core of who we are. Understanding is the only way you can get someone to let go of something they hold dear. We used to think the world was flat. Had we merely been told it was round (not flat) I doubt any of us would have been convinced. People had to sail around the world (without falling off) and gravity had to be explained before we reluctantly exchanged our map for a globe. Same goes for food. For those of you still counting calories and fat grams, I hope to give you enough proof to change your beliefs about food and nutrition.

FAT, OUR FABULOUS FRIEND

Unlike the other two macronutrients, protein and carbohydrates, I would venture to say that fat is the only one you can happily eat by itself. You may feel that you are a carbohydrate addict, but aren't those carbs just a delivery system for something else? That bread becomes great when you spread something on it, potatoes are dull on their own, and who eats pasta without a sauce?

Even the proteins usually need a little help. Chicken and fish are both bland without adding some flavor, and I doubt you would want a burger with nothing but the meat inside the bun.

Fat, however, can go naked and alone. Whole eggs, cheese, nuts, cream, and avocado can all go solo. Fat is our fabulous, flavorful friend and we were denied it for decades.

Another word for fat is "lipid". A lipid molecule is a fat like molecule that cannot dissolve in water.

Fat is more energy dense than carbohydrates and protein. Carbohydrates and protein have four calories per gram. Fat has nine calories per gram and this scared the hell out of us for half a century. So, fat has more calories (energy) than protein or carbohydrates; this might be of concern if we eat the same quantity of fats as we do other foods. However, we are not likely to substitute a large bowl of pasta with a large bowl of cream cheese. Nor would we want to swap a potato for the same amount of peanut butter or order a 6oz slab of avocado.

It is true that the energy value of fat is greater than the other two macronutrients, but the reality is we don't eat fat in the same quantities that we eat protein or carbohydrates.

I'm not going to get into the history of how fat got such a bad rap. I will say that there were some dubious studies over 50 years ago that led to some far reaching assumptions.

A DIFFERENT PATH

When we eat fats, they are broken down into single fatty acids just like protein had to be broken down into amino acids.

Fat can be used for energy; fats are needed for the fat soluble vitamins D E K and A. Fat is also the building block for cell membranes, hormones, and brain function.

Every cell we have is surrounded by a cell membrane which is partly comprised of the dietary fat we consume. Optimal health and aging have to do with keeping our cells in good shape. To keep cells healthy, we have to get nutrients and oxygen to them and to do this they have to pass through the fatty membrane surrounding the cell. If we eat good quality fats, that membrane is permeable, and that makes the transportation easy. If that membrane is rigid because of the crappy fats we ate then the cell can become compromised, and this can trigger poor health and disease.

I remember seeing a commercial back in England that spouted "Sugar the fat free food!" I can only guess which industry funded that commercial but with slogans like that it's not surprising that people associated fat on their plate with fat on their body. The 1980s was the decade of fat free obsession, but the ropy idea also survived the 1990s and is not uncommon today.

Ironically, dietary fat is not the most lipogenic nutrient. Lipogenesis is the creation of new fat. If you want to point a finger, then point it at the high fructose corn syrup which has infiltrated our food supply. Fructose (a fruit sugar) is highly lipogenic, but our man made high fructose corn syrup blows natural fructose out of the water when it comes to the body's ability to make body fat.

Fat is good, it can be used for energy, it's needed for hormones, vitamins and every cell in our body. What's more, it tastes good and, especially for the ladies out there, it doesn't hold onto water weight the way that those bread, cereals, and grains do.

Fats can be saturated fats (solid at room temperature), monounsaturated fats and polyunsaturated fats. Most fats are a combination, and their designation falls to the most dominant type of fat present. For example, coconut oil is over 90 percent saturated fat, butter 68 percent saturated fat, olive oil only 14 percent saturated fat.

For those of you who like to cook, it is always best to cook with a highly saturated fat (like coconut oil). Its level of saturation makes it more stable and less likely to go rancid with heat. Again, my grandmother had it right cooking in butter and lard. Avoid cooking with vegetable oils; they are highly processed and high in omega 6, which is linked to inflammation and associated with asthma, depression, heart disease and even some cancers. They can also alter the fat profile in our cells. Avoid Soybean, corn, rapeseed, cottonseed, grapeseed, safflower and rice bran oil; curiously, all classed as vegetable oils and yet none come from the healthy vegetables we are encouraged to eat more of.

When choosing a fat to cook with, look for unprocessed, natural oils like coconut oil, animal fats (lard and tallow), for shallow frying you can use olive oil, palm oil and avocado oil (similar to olive oil). For lengthier cooking times it's best to avoid butter because it contains trace amounts of protein and carbohydrates, which can then burn.

THE FAT BREAKDOWN

"Triglycerides" are the form of fat stored in your body. Body fat is made up of triglycerides. To break down the word triglyceride, "tri" meaning "three", identifies that there are three fatty acids. "Glycerides" denotes that the three individual fatty acids are connected to glycerol. So, a triglyceride is three fatty acids and a glycerol unit. Triglycerides are made by the body and come from the foods that we eat.

When we are talking about the differences in fat, we are talking about the differences in the three fatty acids that make up a triglyceride.

The fat in the foods we eat can be saturated, monounsaturated, polyunsaturated and they can be the chemically altered trans fats.

SATURATED FAT

Saturated fat has no carbon carbon double bonds (see diagram). Because there are no bonds, this fat is referred to as saturated and includes dairy products, cheeses and meats.

Saturated fats are easily identified as they are solid at room temperature. In the past, saturated fats were thought to increase the risk of coronary heart disease, but this has been strongly challenged. We still have a hung jury on the fate of saturated fat with strong advocates on either side of the argument. However, it seems safe to assert that saturated fat is not the extreme villain we once thought it was.

Natural foods contain a combination of fats, and their designation is based on which is most dominant.

For example, coconut oil is classed as a saturated fat because it is 90% saturated fat. Butter is 64% saturated and lard comes in at 40% saturated.

Foods that are classed as saturated fats are coconut oil, milk fat, pork fat (lard), butter, cream and chicken and beef fat.

When a fat does have one carbon carbon double bond, it is,

unsurprisingly, called a "monounsaturated fat" because "mono" means "one".

Saturated Fat

Monounsaturated Fat

Polyunsaturated Fat

Don't let the memory of high school chemistry scare you. All you have to understand is there is one double bond in monounsaturated fat, and that makes it different from saturated fat.

MONOUNSATURATED FAT

If there are still some doubters when it comes to how healthy saturated fat is, we can have a clear conscience when it comes to monounsaturated fats.

Monounsaturated fats are found in red meat, avocados, olives, oil (hazelnuts, olives, safflowers, peanuts, etc.), nuts and fish. Monounsaturated fats are thought by everyone to be the "healthy fats".

While "mono" means one, "poly" of course means more than one.

POLYUNSATURATED FATS

Polyunsaturated fats contain more than one carbon carbon double bonds. The two most common polyunsaturated fats are omega 3 and omega 6. I am sure you've heard these names kicked around. The '3' simply refers to the position of the last carbon carbon double bond in the fatty acids chain.

Polyunsaturated fats are found in seeds, nuts, certain meats and significantly in fish. Polyunsaturated fats, just like monounsaturated fats, get a unanimous thumbs up and are definitely among the hallowed "healthy fats".

When we talk about "healthy fats" we are referring to naturally occurring fats from both animal and plant sources. Where it all goes wrong is when money gets involved, and we start talking big business, economies of scale, competition and supply and demand.

Fat tastes great and is included in a great many products, and yet those products can only sell if they can last the test of time, meaning survive long haul transportation and endure an extended shelf life. Fish, meats, dairy and the innocent avocado don't stand a chance against the fats used in fast foods, cakes, pastries and other tempting processed foods.

TRANSFATS

I would like to think by the time I finish this book that trans fats will be a nonissue. I would like to think that the USA will follow the lead set by other countries in banning these fats.

Remember that saturated fats are stable and solid because they do not contain any double bonds. Now, hydrogenation is the process that removes double bonds from polyunsaturated fats and in so doing converts them into single bonds. Predictably, this process converts liquids into solids and produces "hydrogenated" fats.

You do not have to understand the image below. Just note that it is dissimilar to the other natural fat profiles.

"Trans" fatty acid

"Partially hydrogenated fats" is a statement you will often see on the labels of foods. This just means the hydrogenation process was not completed. Trans fats are these partially hydrogenated fats; they do contain double bonds, but not in a way that is found in nature.

The word "trans" refers to a different configuration of the double bonds. This might be starting to sound a little confusing, but all you need to know is this: when you see "trans fat" or "partially hydrogenated" it means the fat has been artificially altered and is undeniably linked to an increased risk of cardiovascular disease.

The jury is unanimous in its verdict here, and trans fats are guilty as all hell. They should be avoided at all times. The sure fire way to avoid these processed fats is merely to avoid processed foods. Thankfully, processed foods do require a label so if you can't avoid them altogether, then please read the label and watch out for the words "trans fats" and the deceiving term "partially hydrogenated fat/oil".

If you feed a rabbit (an herbivore, a plant eater) cholesterol (animal derived) rich foods and fat, and that rabbit gets heart disease should we base medical guidelines around the observation of a rabbit forced to eat non rabbit foods? NO, and yet that is what happened, and people were told not to eat fat for fear of risking the fate that befell the rabbits.

It was said that polyunsaturated fats (made from crops) were good for the heart and people like my mom switched from real butter and lard to margarine, a highly processed product which emerged in the 1970s.

Some would point out that margarine popularity was partly due to the heavily funded Heart Association which favored the crop industry. Others would say studies were just inaccurately read and poor assumptions were made. However, we got there, we moved away from raw, natural fats and into an era of heavily processed polyunsaturated and trans fats.

Dietary fat has been nutrition's greatest victim and only now are we dusting it down and appreciating its true glory.

Nuts

- Walnuts

- Almonds

- Cashews

- Hazelnuts

- Macadamia

- Pistachio

- Pecans

- Peanuts (legume)

Also, the above as nut butter (be very careful to read the label as often full of sugar)

Oils

- Coconut Oil (great choice for cooking to cook)

- Olive Oil

- Avocado

- Flaxseed

- Walnut oil

- Avoid all vegetable oils

Also

- Egg Yolks

- Butter (not margarine) raw is best

- Avocado

- Cheese

- Guacamole (read the label)

- Sour Cream

- Full fat milk and cream

- Salad Dressings (read the label)

- Sesame and Flaxseed

- Fish Oil as a supplement (Omega 3 fatty acid) and cod liver or Krill oil

ANIMAL FATS

The fattier meats are considered to be those with more than 4.5 grams of saturated fat in a single serving of 100 grams

Found in our non lean protein choices

- Fatty cuts of beef including T bone and ribs

- Fatty fish (salmon, anchovies, Sea Bass, Carp, Eel, Herring, sardines, white fish)

- Chicken thigh (other poultry and poultry skin)

For those who would like to join the dots, let's discuss how the fat on your plate ends up being used by your body.

Fat is very different from the other two macronutrients, protein, and carbohydrates, in that nothing happens to fat until it reaches the small intestine. Carbohydrates start getting broken down in the mouth when we chew and secrete salivary enzymes, and protein, although not broken down in the mouth, starts disassembling when it is in the stomach.

Fat passes unscathed from the mouth, down the esophagus, and through the stomach until it reaches the small intestine. This is why fat keeps us feeling full; when that fat is in our stomach there is no digestion taking place, so we feel full/satiated. Foods that are described as "rich" or "heavy" are usually high fat foods. Perhaps

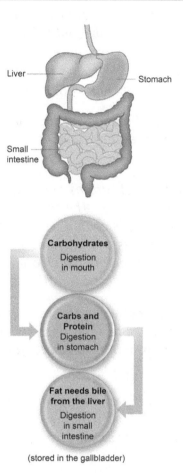

Liver — Stomach

Small intestine —

Carbohydrates
Digestion in mouth

Carbs and Protein
Digestion in stomach

Fat needs bile from the liver
Digestion in small intestine

(stored in the gallbladder)

you've been in a fancy French restaurant where the meal came out, and it was tiny. You think to yourself, how you're going to have to eat again afterwards because this so called portion is so small. Then you eat... and feel full. Yes, it's the high fat protein and sauces the French are famous for; rich and heavy with fat. It's also the reason that low fat meals tend to leave you feeling hungry.

Frozen yogurt is a big hit with the low fat brigade. I would go to this one place in West LA and there would be these ultra thin ladies glugging their gallon sized fat free yogurts. They would never dare eat a regular yogurt of the same size; they would be scared to death of the calories, but also a full fat yogurt of that same size would have you feeling so full I doubt you could finish it.

Fat travels a long way before the body gets to work on breaking it down. Bile (made in the liver) mixes with fat in the small intestine. Bile salts emulsify the fat into smaller droplets, and now pancreatic lipase (fat digesting enzyme) can do its job and further break fat down into free fatty acids and monoglycerides.

These free fatty acids and monoglycerides are packaged together into triglycerides (remember these?) while in the lining of the small intestine.

Whereas protein and carbohydrates enter the blood supply from the small intestine, fat does not. The fat, now packaged together into its transportable form, is coated with protein and lipids, and can travel in water. The fats are now known as lipoproteins and enter the lymphatic system before heading upward to a big vein in your neck where they at long last enter the blood supply.

The lymphatic system is a network of tubes mapping the entire body. It drains fluid from tissue, filters out bacteria, is home to infection fighting white blood cells and it transports fatty acids before they enter the general blood supply.

Bacteria, filtered out of the body during illness, is stored in the lymph nodes. You may have experienced the swelling of these lymph nodes at times when you have been sick.

> Dietary fat takes longer to be broken down.
>
> It has to be re-packaged before it can travel and it travels first in the lymph system before entering your blood system.

THE EXCEPTION TO THE RULE

You can live a good life without knowing the journey of fat but here is an exception you might hear bandied about a lot, especially if you live the low carb life.

Most of your dietary fats are "long chain triglycerides" just think literally... a long chain of fat. There are also a few "medium chain triglycerides"... yes, a shorter chain of fat.

The medium chain triglycerides (MCT) are digested like carbohydrates. They are absorbed into the small intestine and enter the bloodstream directly (they do not travel via the lymphatic system) and then go to your liver where they can be used for fuel. This is a major difference!

MCT's became an iconic supplement when the low carb diets first hit. Because they enter the bloodstream faster, you can get energy /fuel like you would from a carbohydrate. For those choosing to eat very low carbohydrate, MCT's are an excellent choice.

Although the supplement industry makes buckets of money from MCT products, you can find them right on your grocery store shelves in the form of coconut oil, palm kernel oil, and whole milk

If you want to give your low carb diet a kick, load up on your MCTs.

CARBOHYDRATES, THE BAD RELATIONSHIP WE CAN'T KICK

If you are numb from the last two macronutrients, hold on as the ride is about to change. If there's one macronutrient we are expected to understand beyond all others, it is carbohydrates. If you've ever tried to lose weight in the last ten years, you will have tried to limit your carbohydrate intake. I would suggest that most of the people trying to cut their carbohydrates have no idea why.

The conversation goes something like this

Question   Why don't you eat carbohydrates?

Answer   "They make me fat" or

or   "The make me bloated" or

or   "My body is super sensitive to carbs"

Question   Why is that?

Answer   .... ?

I almost called this book "Beyond the Second Why" because few people understand their relationship with carbohydrates beyond that initial first response.

If you are paying someone money for their nutritional guidance and they can't answer beyond the second, why then please ask for your money back and run away.

The weight loss industry is terrible for this. They tell people "Don't eat carbs", sell them products but don't explain a thing.

People who tried to lose weight in the 1970's were terrified of calories. Anyone trying to lose weight today is terrified of carbohydrates. The sadness is when they succumb to the calories or binge on the carbs that person feels terrible about themselves. Self loathing creeps in which leads to feelings of failure and defeat.

I had a client, a successful guy whose weight continually went up and down. He lost weight by counting calories and starving himself. He would ask how many calories we had burned in a workout so that he could estimate his calories perfectly, intake and output. I met with him for nutrition many times and created meal plans yet. Still, every year he would starve himself down the scale and then rebound right back up.

One day I asked him about his fascination with calories, and he told me that he had once had a trainer who was in incredible shape. This trainer had told my client that he just made sure he didn't ever eat more than 1500 calories per day. This little gem had stuck with my client. It made sense; the information came from a credible source and a source that my client could relate to (male, about the same age and with a physique my guy admired).

A little hurt that my hours of teaching had been ignored due to a one liner from another trainer, I asked my client when he had been told this. "Over twenty years ago," he replied. He had held on to this comment about calories per day for over two decades! He had tried and failed for over twenty years to limit his daily calorie intake, and overall, he was getting heavier and heavier with each passing year.

I saw how to break the belief my client had formed about fat loss. When he told me that the comment had been made over twenty years, I told my client that I would have likely given him the same advice... twenty years ago.

I suggested that if he contacted that trainer today he would not be given the same answer.

This (at long last) struck a chord. We spent time discussing nutrition and weight loss again, but this time my client was present and receptive. He immediately started dropping weight without starving himself. Today he is 30lb lighter, and he has sustained this new weight for more than two years.

My point here is that I ask you to put on hold any beliefs you have about weight loss and, especially for this next section, about carbohydrates.

I will also say that carbohydrates can make you fat, but that is like saying a brick will break your toe; it will, but only if you drop the brick on your toe. If you eat carbohydrates mindfully, they serve a great purpose as the primary fuel source for your body. If you treat them mindlessly, they are most certainly the one macronutrient that will pack on pounds and add inches.

"CARBS"

Carbohydrates are your rice, pasta, potatoes, bread, cereal, candy bar, cake and pastries, your noodles, fries and tortilla chips as well as your fruit and vegetables. They never come from an animal source, and most of those mentioned are not natural carbohydrates; rather, they are products made from naturally occurring carbohydrates.

There are many words used interchangeably to talk about a carbohydrate; sugar, monosaccharide, disaccharide, glucose, glycogen, fiber, carbs and net carbs. Let's unravel this before we go any further.

A "sugar" is a carbohydrate that can dissolve in water. You can recognize a sugar because it will end in "ose." Food labels may say dextrose, sucralose, maltose, xylose and, of course, high fructose corn syrup, but it all means "sugar"

Carbohydrates are made up of single sugar molecules (a molecule is just a small particle made up of atoms).

A single sugar molecule has six carbon atoms and is called a monosaccharide (mono meaning one, saccharide meaning sugar).

Monosaccharide, therefore, means one sugar particle, so they are often referred to as "Simple Sugars".

MONOSACCHARIDES

- Fructose sugars found in fruit

- Galactose sugars found in mammals' milk

- Glucose you'll hear the word glucose a lot; this is because glucose is the form of sugar your body can use for fuel

When you eat carbohydrates, they must be broken down into single units of sugar – monosaccharides – before they can enter the blood.

DISACCHARIDES

In chemistry, the prefix "di" is used to denote two, double or twice. When talking about carbohydrates, a disaccharide is simply two monosaccharides.

- Sucrose = glucose + fructose (your table sugars, sugar cane, the carbs in fruit and vegetables)

- Lactose = glucose + galactose (found in milk and dairy produce)

- Maltose = glucose + glucose (barley, "malt" sugar)

Disaccharides, because they are made of two monosaccharides, still have to be broken down into the single units of glucose before they can be used. Some people have difficulty breaking down milk sugar lactose and suffer discomfort, gas and bloating as a result. We would say that these people are "lactose intolerant".

OLIGOSACCHARIDES

"Oligo" means "few" so oligosaccharides are three to ten monosaccharides (single sugars) joined together in a chain.

A carbohydrate chain must be broken down into individual units of glucose before it can be used. Part of the oligosaccharide chain cannot be broken and remains undigested. The undigested part has been found to provide healthy bacteria in the colon and reduce the number of unhealthy gut bacteria.

Slightly sweet to the taste, this carbohydrate is gaining interest as a "functional food". It is found in plants, vegetables, breast milk and especially in chicory root, onions, legumes, asparagus and Jerusalem artichokes. Expect to hear more about oligosaccharides as the marketing madness catches wind of something new to shake in your face. It's a great sounding word which makes it seem very important and complex.

Carbohydrates are chains of sugar and oligosaccharides are longer than the two piece chain of a disaccharide but not as long as a polysaccharide.

POLYSACCHARIDES

You are probably noticing the progression; mono (one) di (two) oligo (few) and now poly meaning "many". These chains have more than ten parts to them and can be very long.

The shorter chained carbohydrates are sweeter whereas the polysaccharides are tasteless and, because of a great many bonds/links in their chains, they do not dissolve in water. This is why we sweeten our tea with honey, not broccoli. Honey (glucose+ fructose = disaccharide, sweet and soluble) Broccoli (Polysaccharide, not at all sweet and won't do much of anything in your tea).

You may you have heard of "starchy" carbohydrates? You may have been told to stay away from "starches". Well, starches are one type of polysaccharides. They are long chains of glucose found in root vegetables, potatoes, and cereals. Starchy foods include rice, bread, and pasta, making starch the most popular polysaccharide.

Cellulose is found in the structure of plants. We know it better as fiber. We cannot break down its bonds, and therefore we cannot digest it. Animals, however, can break down and digest cellulose, which is why horses eat hay and we probably shouldn't.

Pectin is a polysaccharide found in plant roots and fruits. Apples are the best known source of pectin. In water, it forms a gel and can be used as a setting agent or a glaze. It is popular among vegans as an alternative to the animal based gelatin.

Pectin is used for jams and jellies. It is a stabilizer which is also found in bread and even cornflakes. Naturally, pectin is found in all fruits, especially apples, apricots, grapefruits, and oranges. Pectin is also found in vegetables, especially colorful carrots and tomatoes.

Sources of pectin are popular because, as a type of soluble fiber, pectin slows the passage of food thereby slowing the release of glucose into your blood. This is a good thing. The final polysaccharide we will discuss is glycogen. If you work out you may be familiar with the terms; glycogen, glycogen storage, glycogen uptake, glycogen depletion. These fancy terms merely refer to the storage form of glucose. We can store the carbohydrates that we eat in our muscles.

Glycogen is found in our muscles, liver, and brain. When carbohydrates are broken down into single units of glucose they can then enter the blood. From the blood, glucose can be used for immediate fuel or it can be stored for future fuel. Glucose stored in muscle, the liver or the brain is called glycogen. We have about a day's worth of fuel stored as glycogen.

Carbohydrates are all "sugar" and "sugar" is not a bad word.

Carbohydrates are energy foods that come from the sun hitting a plant.

Carbohydrates can be formed under ground, above ground or even up a tree.

Carbohydrates can be long or short chains of sugar units. The longer chains are called "complex," and the shorter chains are called "simple".

All chains are broken down into single units of glucose which enter the bloodstream and can be used as fuel immediately or stored as future fuel.

There are a great many confusing terms that basically describe the same thing. We hear about simple sugars and starches; we talk about complex carbs and glucose. Fructose is demonized, and yet honey is idolized. Sugar is to be avoided, and we are told to stick to the "good" carbohydrates, yet now we know that all carbohydrates are sugar. It all gets very confusing.

FIBER

So where does fiber fit in? We are told to eat more of it in the form of vegetables and whole grains. "Whole grains" is another term thrown around with cheerful abandon, conjuring up a picture of a "wholesome" hunk of unsliced bread. Just for the record, you don't have to eat any grains to get enough fiber in your day.

Food cannot enter the bloodstream in the form in which it lies on your plate. We don't have a piece of chicken or a bagel floating around in our blood. Food is broken down by the digestive system into an absorbable/usable form:

Protein is broken down into amino acids.

Fat is broken down into fatty acids.

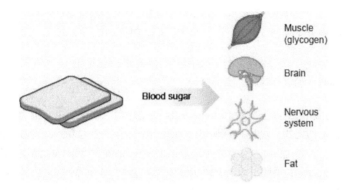

Carbohydrates are broken down into single units of glucose.

Fiber, in contrast, is not broken down and if something we eat cannot be broken down it is not digested and therefore not absorbed into our bloodstream.

Although fiber never enters our blood it has immense health benefits. When we think of bacteria we think of invisible dirt coating innocent surfaces. It lurks on grocery cart handles, in bathroom stalls ,and on gym equipment. We avoid it, wiping down that grocery cart, carefully placing seat covers on a public toilet and wearing gloves and carrying towels in the gym. Our body, however, is full of bacteria. We have more bacterial than we do human cells. We are talking hundreds of different types, and trillions of cells in total. There are both good and bad bacteria, so we focus on not picking up the bad stuff that makes us sick.

There are plenty of good bacteria, mostly living in our guts. Think of your "gut" as your digestive tract, or simply whether the food goes after you eat it. It goes to your stomach and then on to your small intestine, into your large intestine and then exits your body.

Just as we need to eat to survive, so do cells and bacteria. Cells are fed when the food that we eat is digested and absorbed into our bloodstream, after which nutrients can travel to cells. This is where fiber enters the story. Fiber cannot be digested because our gut does not have the necessary enzymes to break it down – that's why we need bacteria.

Fiber passes through the stomach and the small intestine unchanged. When it reaches the large intestine bacteria will get to work breaking it down and feeding upon it. This is how fiber works as a "prebiotic".

Prebiotics are the food for probiotics and probiotics are the good bacteria we were talking about in the first place.

These probiotics are associated with a great many health benefits. Fiber feeds good bacteria in the gut and this is a very good thing. What is not so great is the bloating and gas it can create. When bacteria feed on fiber it produces gas. And it is this gas that can cause bloating and it is this gas that embarrasses women and turns men into seven year old boys.

There are two types of fiber: soluble and insoluble.

Soluble fiber dissolves in water and becomes gel like. This is the fiber that expands our stomach by dragging in the water and creating more bulk. Insoluble fiber does not dissolve in water. Most foods that contain fiber will have both soluble and insoluble fiber.

Fiber does not enter our bloodstream. Its purpose lies with intestinal health. As a ballpark we should aim to eat 30 40g of fiber per day.

Fiber travels straight through our body doing a lot of good deeds along the way but it never enters our bloodstream.

The mono, di, oligo and polysaccharides do end up in the blood and can be used as fuel or can be placed in storage.

Carbohydrates start getting broken down with our first bite. The saliva in our mouth has enzymes that start the process and give us that sweet tasting delight of the first bite. The carbohydrates travel down your esophagus (throat area) into your stomach and on to your small intestine. It is here in the small intestine (duodenum) that they really get acted upon, by pancreatic amylase. The pancreas is positioned near the small intestine and enzymes travel from the pancreas to the small intestine to aid digestion.

Whatever form the carbohydrate was in when it started off – maybe it was a bagel, the carbs in a candy bar or a sandwich – it is now in the form of monosaccharides; the single units of sugar that pass through the wall of the small intestine and enter our blood.

Once in the blood we can call these carbohydrates "blood sugar" or "blood glucose". They travel in the blood to the liver. The liver processes and then repackages or eliminates anything you ate or drank (this includes medications and alcohol) before sending it back into the general blood supply via the hepatic vein.

As you understand the journey of food, you can see how that journey is affected by health. If we have digestive issues affecting the small intestine, or pancreatic issues affecting the enzymes and hormones it releases, or a liver disease, food can become a problem for the body instead of effective nourishment.

If you have a food allergy, then you know all too well how this feels.

> Protein and fat have numerous functions, from making hormones, enzymes and muscles to protecting cells and our network of nerves. Carbohydrates, on the other hand, have one main job to do; fuel the body, brain, nervous system and red blood cells that carry the all-important oxygen.
>
> How much carbohydrate can be stored in our muscles is limited by how much lean body mass we have. Bittersweet is the unlimited capacity for excess carbohydrates to be taken via the liver and stored in fat cells.

Let's say you are lactose intolerant and are not able to digest dairy: it doesn't matter how healthy that raw unpasteurized $10 a carton organic cream is, it will pass through you undigested, doing you no good and causing hours of discomfort.

CARBOHYDRATE STORAGE

The carbohydrates not immediately used for fuel can be stored as 'glycogen'. The liver can store a little bit of glycogen but, although the liver is quite a large organ and a big hitter in the organ world, it really doesn't like to store much glycogen, maybe a few hundred calories. However, what we really rely on for glycogen storage is our muscles.

The more muscle we have, the more carbohydrates we can store as glycogen. That might mean a thousand or several thousand calories worth of carbohydrates, depending on how much muscle you have. How much we store in muscles also depends on how active the muscle is; conditioned athletes having the ability to store a lot more glycogen than most people.

Beware: once carbohydrates enter a muscle they remain there until that muscle uses that 'glycogen' as energy. This is critical if you want to lose weight. If you find yourself sedentary for any reason you will not deplete your muscles' glycogen stores. If you eat an excess of carbohydrates, the muscles stores will max out and those carbohydrates will show up as body fat.

Dealing with this fact depends on circumstance. If, for example, you are sick in the hospital you may need carbohydrates to heal, so you cannot just cut them out. By contrast, if you're on vacation, resting your butt on a beach lounger for a week, you may want to reconsider that dessert they're offering you. If your muscles are not active, then that dessert is going straight to that thing you're sitting on.

- There is a limit to how many carbohydrates can be stored in muscle.

- Stored carbohydrates are called glycogen

- Glycogen will only fuel the muscle it is in. Only liver glycogen can travel and fuel the rest of the body.

With this in mind, consider the concept of "carbing up"; an age old practice of eating massive amounts of carbohydrates before an event. The story goes this will give you energy and fuel.

If you can only store X amount of carbohydrates, what is the point of eating 10 x that amount? Where is the excess meant to go? I'll give you one guess.

Over the years I have met with many clients who came to see me because they gained weight getting ready for an endurance event. The amount of carbohydrates they were told to eat is always the reason why.

To make a bad story even worse...

Carbohydrates are transported into muscle by the hormone insulin. When we eat a high carbohydrate meal our blood sugar increases and triggers insulin. The body dislikes high levels of sugar in the blood and its insulin's job to get rid of it. When blood sugar is high insulin will not only transport the carbohydrates out of our blood, but it will also lock fat in our fat cells. It makes good sense that insulin traps one source of fuel while it deals with an abundance of another.

When we are working out insulin is inhibited, which also makes good sense, as we want to keep carbohydrates in the blood to travel to the muscles being used. Glut4 is the transporter that takes sugar from the blood to the working muscles while we are exercising. When the muscle is dormant glut4 is not active and we rely again on insulin to remove sugar from the blood. The kicker here is that it takes a "boatload" of insulin to get carbohydrates into a known active muscle. If insulin can't get the carbohydrates into the muscle where does it end up? In fat cells.

I'm sure you've heard the Old Wives Tale, "Don't eat before bedtime!"

They should be saying, "Don't eat carbohydrates at night."

The most relaxed part of the day for most people is the evening. Sitting on the couch watching TV or trolling social media. Not the ideal time to order pizza or to eat cookies or pasta. Your muscles are rested, and it would take a lot of insulin to get any of those carbs into your inactive muscles. If the carbs cannot travel to muscles, they will end up in fat.

If you eat enough carbohydrates to elicit a huge insulin response, then insulin will do its job and trap fat in fat cells.

If you're trying to lose weight skip the carbs at night and stick to protein, fat and vegetables. If you're working out in the evening, then you can disregard the Old Wives Tale altogether because your muscles are active and receptive and ready to store more carbohydrates.

The carbohydrates your muscles store are the fuel you need for your next workout, which brings me on to another gem.

"Eat before your workout to fuel your workout."

You wake up and have a hearty carb rich breakfast in preparation for your workout.

The fear is if you don't have that breakfast you won't have the energy or strength to get through your training session.

Knowing what you know now does it make sense to have that breakfast? You just woke up, so the muscles are not active, they are not primed to take on those pancakes but not to worry, your fat cells will oblige.

I suggested skipping breakfast to a dear cardiologist friend of mine who trains in the morning. He dropped 15lb.

In the summer of 2010 a gentleman came to see me at my nutrition office in Santa Monica and he was pretty upset as he had just dedicated six months of his life to transforming himself from (his words) "a lifelong coach potato" into a man who ran the LA Marathon. He ran with a running group and had a goal to raise money for a charity close to his heart and also to lose the weight he had been gaining since he turned 40.

He completed the marathon, raised the money and gained ten pounds.

He sat in my office furious, accusatory, even though this was my first time meeting him. He left the office understanding why he had gained weight and with a plan to correct it. His coaches had encouraged that hearty breakfast and a heavy carb diet. He was still furious but at least it was no longer directed at me. I think he was heading straight to the running club that had told him to eat bagels and bananas for breakfast.

Please know that even the most well intentioned coach or exercise instructor may be giving outdated advice.

Another gentleman came to see me in the fall of 2015. He had lost a lot of weight, over 80 pounds, and he had kept the weight off for five years until he suffered an injury and had to limit his exercise greatly. I asked him how he had lost weight initially and he said from becoming very active and watching his portion size. This was a guy who had hiked every local elevation possible, in between grueling ultra marathons. He lost weight not because his nutrition was the best (it was not) but because he was exercise reliant and continually in a state of muscle glycogen depletion. In other words, he was continually depleting the glycogen stored in his muscles so that he always had storage room for the carbohydrates he was still over consuming. When he got injured the exercise stopped and on came the weight. He had quickly regained almost all 80 pounds.

When you have somebody with that sort of discipline, it's an easy fix. We merely restructured the way he ate his macronutrients, and he started to lose weight again. A few months later his injuries had all healed and he was back to his intense workouts, but this time he wasn't relying on excessive exercise to keep him in shape.

In the 1970s we focused on calories if we wanted to lose weight. In the 1980s we focused on fat free foods. In the 90s we started to learn more about the role of carbohydrates and body composition. It's all got obsessive, confusing and contradictory, prioritizing the calories, the fat grams or the carbohydrates and now, as we barrel towards 2020, we are becoming fearful of meat. There are sgenuine concerns about how animals are fed and treated, and we are entering an era of conscious and ethical living, but more of that anon.

CHAPTER TWO: BODY FAT

SECTION 1: BODY FAT

I have rolls. If you want to find my fat, just pinch me. These lovely rolls sit around my waist and on my back. My fat is 'subcutaneous' meaning that it lies under the skin for all to pinch! I do not have the typical female fat patterning. Most women have smaller waists and hold fat on their butt, hips, and thighs, often giving a nice curvy look. No, this is not me. My legs are slim, and my hips narrow; you may see me in shorts but never in a belly shirt.

Body fat is stored in different ways and zoned differently between men and women. As I say, the rolls I have are of subcutaneous fat. Other people, especially women, often have 'intramuscular triglycerides' (IMTG) and their fat is stored in the muscle. Imagine a slab of meat. Some meat has the fat layer on the top (that would be me) and is the type of fat you may ask the butcher to trim off, whereas other meat has a marbled effect, with fat running throughout. That is IMTG (intramuscular triglycerides).

IMTGs, in my opinion, are more attractive. It is those curvy ladies, the girls with solid butts and thighs but not a roll to be seen, the girls you see in music videos with the tiny waists, curvy behinds, and shapely legs. Their fat is within the muscle which means you cannot pinch it. It is the same fat that some women confuse with muscle. They mistakenly think they have heavily muscled thighs; in most cases, it is muscle full of fat.

I have known ladies that don't want to train legs because they think their legs are muscular enough already. In most cases, the reality is that they are holding fat in their legs which makes them look big. It would be a real mistake NOT to train that area because that lower body fat is not going anywhere unless it is burnt up as fuel. The fear of their legs getting even bigger is unfounded because if the exercise uses some of that fat for fuel, their trained legs will most certainly get smaller.

IMTGs show up in women as heavier triceps, solid hips and butt and thighs that dominate. Overall, I might have less fat than these women, but these ladies have a much sexier way of carrying any excess.

The ultimate test is the flex test. If you flex your thigh muscles and you don't see any separation, then what you are looking at is fat. The muscle may appear to be rock hard, but if there are no lines to show the different muscles of the thigh, then you are looking at fat. On the other hand, if you flex your legs and you can see all sorts of detail going on, then you are looking at some beautiful, lean muscular legs.

It is the people with the IMTGs that I have difficulty measuring for body fat using standard calipers. The calipers measure the thickness of the skin, and if your fat is underneath the skin like mine, then it's a simple measurement to take. When a person's fat is in the muscle, I cannot pinch it using calipers, and the reading is often inaccurate. For this reason, I also use an ultrasound device that can measure body fat held in muscle.

Visceral fat. This is the dangerous fat that has a strong link to heart disease. Visceral fat wraps itself around the organs and makes for a protruding midsection. It's the guy with the 42 inch waist that proudly lifts his shirt to show how firm his "abs" are, proudly he slaps them declaring, "It's all muscle, baby."

I can see how the confusion arises as the midsection is indeed solid and you would expect fat to be soft and squishy, but a 42 inch waistline with 18 inch thighs is neither healthy nor attractive. If your waist measurement is greater than your hip measurement, it is a reason to be concerned, rolls or no rolls.

This visceral abdominal fat is associated with an increased risk of high blood pressure, high cholesterol, coronary heart disease, type II diabetes and premature death.

So, we have subcutaneous fat (SQ fat), easy to see, easy to measure and hard to ignore. We have intramuscular triglycerides (IMTG), the fat stored within the muscle, can look sexy, is hard to pinch and often mistaken for lean mass. Thirdly, visceral fat that wraps around the organs making for a turtle belly often joked about but far from funny due to its known relationship with heart disease.

One more place we find fat is in our blood. The liver makes fat and releases it into the blood as triglycerides (TG). You may have seen it in the results from a blood test. It is important to know how much fat is in your blood as this may indicate a necessary nutritional adjustment. High triglycerides can show that you are eating too many carbs because an excess of carbohydrates will be turned into fat by the liver.

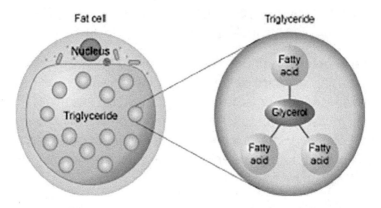

Triglycerides are the storage form of fat. As the name suggests, TRI GLYcerides are comprised of 3 fatty acids and 1 unit of glycerol.

SECTION 2: BODY SHAPE & BODY TYPES

BODY SHAPE

Our body shape is dependent on our bone structure and on where our fat decides to take up residence. Fat patterning is firstly a matter of gender. Men hold more upper body fat, especially on their torso, back, waistline and chest. Women seem to have a broader range when it comes to body shape, from the very estrogenic body to the very androgenic body.

Estrogenic women, at one end of the spectrum, are usually shorter, bustier, have small waists and larger hips and thighs. At the other end of the spectrum is the more androgenic shape. These women are taller, have smaller busts and blockier waistlines with comparatively slim hips and thighs. The estrogenic women usually have rounder faces, whereas the androgenic women have squarer jaws. These are two opposite ends of the spectrum, and in between lies all manner of variation. I have a much more androgenic, straight up and down physique (with rolls).

I can eat well and train hard, but I will never create the curves of Shakira or the Kardashian clan. Likewise, they could spend their fortunes and never have my boyish lines although I doubt that would be a good business move for any of them.

Identify with your body shape and how you hold fat, own it and get over any hang ups you might have. Be the best version of yourself and don't compare yourself to others. If you need someone to aspire to please pick someone who has the same body type and fat patterning as you. You will be continually frustrated is you idolize a body type that is not your own.

BODY TYPES

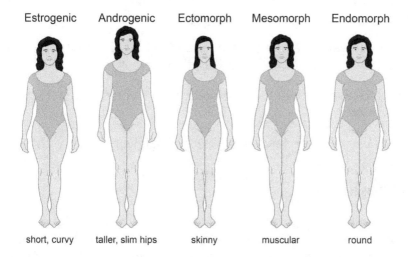

| Estrogenic | Androgenic | Ectomorph | Mesomorph | Endomorph |
| short, curvy | taller, slim hips | skinny | muscular | round |

There are three classic body types that apply to both men and women.

1. ECTOMORPH

This is the person who seemingly can eat what they want and never gain weight. They have a lighter frame and very few curves. A true ectomorph will have slightly pointy facial features, long fingers, and fine hair. Ironically, they are often very active or hyperactive people. Infuriatingly, with no noticeable weight issue, they tend to love exercise. It's the skinny chick that runs eight miles a day or that annoying guy in the office that's still full of life well after 5.00 pm.

Ectomorphs get minimal sympathy when they complain about their weight, but in their defense when they do hold the weight it is in their midsection. Lift their shirts, and they have a little pouch of fat that drives them mad. When they try to lose weight, they get even skinner, and that pouch stays put.

Ectomorphs are hard gainers it's a real challenge for them to build muscle even though pound for pound they can be extremely strong.

2. MESOMORPH

A Mesomorph can build muscle quite quickly. but they can also gain fat. This is your American football player or almost any strength athlete. A true meso will get great results if their nutrition and training is on point. They have the advantage of being able to build muscle, which increases their metabolic rate and makes fat loss easier.

Meso's can eat pizza and drink beer and get away with it for a little while. It will, however, catch up with them eventually.

If I had to identify myself with a body type, I would consider myself a Mesomorph.

Female Mesomorphs have an athletic build; fewer curves, with more of a boyish figure.

3. ENDOMORPH

Endomorphs can build muscle, but they can also carry a lot of body fat. A true Endomorph will have a rounder face, shorter pudgier fingers and toes, and they have beautiful skin that is less prone to wrinkles. Endo's have a much tougher time losing weight, but it is not impossible. When they do lose the weight, they may appear to be closer to a Mesomorph, but they have a lot less wiggle room and must be diligent if they want to keep the weight off.

Although we have three body types, most people will fall somewhere between two of them. You may identify yourself as an Ecto Meso or Meso Endo These classifications are useful when determining the most effective way to exercise and diet. By identifying with a body type, you can put your focus on the right place. If you are working with a personal trainer or nutritionist, it should be one of the first things they take into account.

The classifications should not be seen as limitations. We all know the Ectomorph/hard gainer that built a killer gym physique, and we all know the Endomorph who dropped the weight revealing a whole new body shape and went on the inspire millions.

Examples

A True Female Ectomorph in her 30s:

This lady needs to lift big weights. She is never going to get "too big" and the muscle she does build will add shape to her small frame. This lady does not need to follow a restrictive diet; her main concern will be the protein necessary to build muscle.

This lady will be conscious of her belly pouch, and a good nutritionist will show her how to time her higher carbohydrate meals around her workouts to allow her to maximize fat burning without sacrificing her muscle gains.

A True Male Endomorph in his 30s:

This guy is concerned about his weight. It would be a mistake to focus his workout time on lifting heavy weights because although he is carrying a fair amount of fat, he probably has a lot of muscle as well.

A good trainer will incorporate more circuit training, with resistance work at a much faster pace. Both moderate intensity and high intensity training will be beneficial when combined with a restriction on carbohydrates. If carbohydrates are allowed, they will be eaten immediately after a workout (see the previous chapter regarding carbohydrate storage).

A True Mesomorph in their 40s, male or female:

These people have enjoyed a carefree time during their 20s and 30s. They worked out, got ecxcellent results and if they gained a few pounds they could sharpen their diet and be back on track in no time.

These blessed individuals can get a wake up call in their 40's.

The athlete that is no longer competing gains weight, and now it's a challenge to get it off. This is a person who has never had to work too hard on their body composition; that identity shift can be a real obstacle for the former athlete.

Some Mesos in their 40s and 50s will find their inner athlete again and soar, while others don't change their eating habits and with less activity, they slide into more of an Endomorph physique.

Former Mesomorphs cling to their identity of years gone by, posting photos 20 years old. It's now that the tortoise beats the hare. The ectomorphs and endomorphs that have been struggling all the while at long last sail past the failing meso proving hard work does pay off.

If you have spent your whole adult life working hard to gain or lose weight you are more equipped to stay in shape than the Mesomorph approaching middle age who suddenly finds they can't button their pants.

A good personal trainer or nutritionist will recognize a (former) Mesomorph and will guide them accordingly. A more balanced nutrition plan with high intensity cardio and resistance training will usually be enough for them to shed the excess pounds. The biggest obstacle here is that identity shift the Mesomorph must come to terms with.

Consider the following:

- How do you store your body fat? (subcutaneous, intramuscular and/or visceral)

- Ladies, are you curvy or are you more straight up and down?

- Ladies and Gentlemen, which body type do you identify with?

SECTION 3: OUR CHANGING BODY SHAPE

As you go through life, your body shape may change. Sex hormones decline, waistlines thicken and ladies as you get past menopause you might find that those thighs you hated slim down. Later in this book, we will discuss the enzyme lipoprotein lipase (LPL), but for now you only have to understand that it helps cells to store fat. When women go through menopause, LPL activity is reduced in the lower body and increased in the upper body, legs slim down while waistlines grow. We know this as 'middle aged spread.' The same goes for men; as they age testosterone decreases and this hormonal shift increases LPL activity in the upper body and fat goes to the chest and waistline.

The hormonal changes during pregnancy promote fat distribution. LPL activity is increased in the lower body, and weight is gained in the butt, hips, and thighs. Once the baby is born, LPL activity decreases in the lower body and increases in the breast tissue.

Another interesting observation is with yo yo dieting; people who diet to lose weight only to regain it and repeat the cycle over and over. This fluctuation in weight leads to an increase in upper body fat. I have seen this a great deal in the fitness industry. Cute young girls with teeny waists do one competition diet after another, and that waist starts to grow. Within just a few years of competing, they are not wearing those bra tops in the offseason anymore.

Ladies with heavy triceps nearly always hold fat in their upper hamstring area. Heavy arms usually mean heavy legs but there might be a tiny waist in between.

Hormones affect weight gain, weight loss, and body shape.

A young girl suffered burns to her lower arm and hand, doctors took skin grafts from her thighs to repair the damage. Thirty years later she had to have liposuction to remove fat from her forearm. This is how powerful hormones are in governing fat distribution.

Fat is itself an organ, wherein hormones are created and stored. We have found at least 19 different hormones in fat. Too much body fat can create a diseased state. A great many health risks can be reduced by shedding excess weight. One example of this is estrogen. There are three types of estrogen. One type of estrogen is found in fat and the more fat you have the more of this estrogen you also have. One form of breast cancer is linked to this estrogen. When we have excess fat, we may be increasing our risk of this cancer because of the increased estrogen.

SECTION 4: BODY FAT IS A GOOD THING?

Fat is future energy; excess nutrients stored in adipose tissue, aka fat. We should be grateful that we save our energy as fat because it doesn't hold on to too much water.

Carbohydrates are also fuel, and they can be stored in our muscle as glycogen. For every unit of glycogen, we hold on to two units of water. When we cut carbohydrates, we use up the glycogen. When the glycogen unit is gone there is nothing to hold the water units. Initially, on a low carb diet, this is the weight loss you see.

If we stored all our energy as carbohydrates, we would also hold a tremendous amount of water. A 165lb person with 20% body fat would weigh over 240lbs if that energy were stored as carbohydrates and not as fat.

Thankfully, there is a limit to how many carbohydrates can be stored in muscle.

SECTION 5: FAT FORMATION

To understand how to lose weight remember that triglycerides are how we store fat. Triglycerides are made up of three molecules of fatty acid with a backbone molecule of glycerol.

Triglycerides are made in adipose tissue, in the liver, and in lactating mammary glands when breastfeeding or immediately after childbirth. They are made by the liver, and travel in the blood; they are stored in adipose tissue. Once in adipose tissue, we sit up and take notice because, as a fat cell holds more triglycerides, our body weight increases and body shape changes.

When we gain weight, we do not necessarily gain fat cells, rather, each cell increases in volume, more lipid is held in each cell. To lose weight we must reduce the volume of each cell.

The number of fat cells we have is established by the time we are young adults. If, during puberty, we increase that number then we face a significant challenge if we try to lose weight as an adult. If you have twice as many fat cells you have to reduce the volume of twice as many fat cells. It is one reason why childhood obesity is so terrifying.

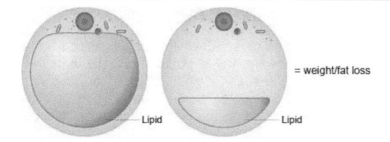

= weight/fat loss

Lipid   Lipid

It is worth noting here that the liver makes fat, but the liver does not like to store fat. 'Fatty liver' refers to a condition when the liver is so overworked it is forced to store fat. This is not meant to happen.

Sadly, we now hear of children with 'fatty liver' an avoidable diseased state.

LIPOGENESIS (NEW FAT)

'Lipogenesis' is the formation of new fat and 'lipolysis' is the breakdown of stored fat. We have many ways to allow for lipogenesis, but the pathway to lipolysis is a lot narrower. There are over 100 known genes that influence fat formation and a list as long as your arm of regulators that push our bodies to store fat. The body has a complete bias in its desire to store fat. Fat is future fuel, and the body needs no encouragement when it comes to creating a stockpile.

You can be storing new fat (lipogenesis), or you can be breaking fat down (lipolysis), but you are not going to be doing both at the same time. Lipogenesis is a cake walk; lipolysis is a tightrope.

You cannot be in two environments at the same time. You cannot be happy and sad at the same time, or tired and energetic. In the same way, you cannot be breaking down stored fat if your body is happily creating new fat.

To win the battle of the bulge, we need to know our competition. We face two intimidating opponents, and our best chance of winning is to know them well. Insulin is a hormone (chemical messenger), and LPL is an enzyme (makes other things happen); if you choose to ignore them you will fail, you will not lose weight.

SECTION 6: INSULIN AND LPL (THE POWERHOUSES)

When we eat food, it is broken down into single units and enters our blood. Carbohydrates are broken down into single units of 'sugar' referred to as "blood sugar" "blood glucose" or simply "sugar." Whether you have just eaten pasta, a burger bun or a bowl of oatmeal, by the time it enters the blood it is all sugar, "blood sugar."

The body dislikes too much glucose in the blood. Blood sugar can become elevated due to:

1. Too many carbohydrates in a meal or drink

2. Meals spaced too closely together

3. A meal that is too large

Blood sugar can get too high by one or a combination of the above, and when there is too much sugar in the blood, it triggers the pancreas to over release the hormone insulin. Insulin is a storage facilitator, and it will transport the glucose out of the blood and into our cells. If it can, it will move glucose into our muscle cells, but it can't always do that. It can, however, get blood sugar into fat cells no problem at all.

Carbohydrates = Insulin = Fat

We do not store fat without the presence of insulin and we have known this for a very long time. Back in the 1930s, insulin was used to treat anorexics; insulin increased hunger and increased fat. On average, patients gained 20lb in their first month.

"Insulin makes us hungry?"

"Don't carbohydrates give us energy?"

Energy bars and workout drinks are full of carbs, and while it is true that glucose is a primary fuel for the brain, nervous system and our cells, glucose itself is not the problem.

Fuel does not equal energy. Too little fuel might make you tired, but excess fuel does not translate to excess energy quite the opposite. The problem is when there is too much glucose, and insulin gets involved. Too many carbohydrates trigger the over release of insulin.

Insulin then does its job and transports the "sugar" out of the blood, ironically now leaving us with low blood sugar and low energy.

High blood sugar can lead to low blood sugar because of insulin.

The perfect example we have all experienced is a food coma. Excess food that leaves us asleep on the couch, not running laps.

That doesn't mean that carbohydrates are off limits. It is "excess" carbohydrates that triggers insulin. If you eat a meal and feel drowsy afterward, you triggered that insulin response.

With the anorexics back in the 1930s, the use of insulin created that drop in blood sugar which in turn created a ferocious appetite as the patient craved carbohydrates to restore blood glucose levels. You do not need to be anorexic to experience this to a slighter degree. The fabulous dinner that you had out last night which led to you feeling drowsy during the drive home and then led to the late night munchies an hour or so later; that was just insulin doing its thing.

Insulin is a hormone, a messenger that travels in the blood and lands on cells which have insulin receptors. A hormone needs its receptor. A key doesn't open every lock and a hormone must lock onto its own receptor to have an effect. Both muscle and fat cells have insulin receptors.

To illustrate the importance of these receptors let's briefly discuss type II diabetes...

Eating a lot of carbohydrates with too little activity leaves the muscle cells full and unable to store anything more. There is a limit to how much they can store and, if we are not active, these stores hit their maximum quickly (within a few thousand calories). Carbohydrates stored in muscle (as glycogen) can be used up with exercise or fasting but if you are inactive and you keep eating then your muscles are going to be full, unable to store anything else, and then where does it all go? Into the fat cells of course.

Michael Phelps might be able to eat 7000 calories a day, the rest of us probably should not.

The person who eats too many carbohydrates without activity will trigger a huge insulin response. Insulin will not be able to get anything into a maxed out muscle cell, but fat cells have no such limits. This person is now getting heavier and even less likely to exercise.

Insulin is a messenger, and the message for the cell is to open up to allow nutrients to be stored. If muscle cells are full they will ignore the message. But insulin doesn't give up, and the pancreas releases even more insulin so that the message gets louder and louder.

Muscle cells eventually tune out insulin and become 'Insulin Resistant'.

Both muscle and fat cells can become insulin resistant, but it will always be the muscle cells that get there first. In extreme cases, the fat cell can also stop listening (this is when the diabetic gets skinny). When cells become resistant, insulin cannot transport nutrients out of the blood. Blood sugar and insulin levels sore to dangerous levels,

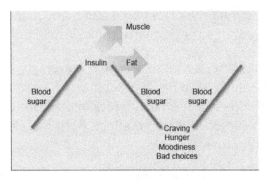

tissue and organs start to become damaged. Diabetics go blind; they lose limbs, they die.

Too much or too little of a hormone is a diseased state.

Insulin is a powerhouse, and we need it, but insulin in itself is not the problem. Some hormones change as we age and some, like insulin, are directly controlled by our own choices and behavior. Take the unborn child for example. It doesn't get to choose its nutrients. In the womb, a child is fed by the circulating blood of the mother, and if the mother has high blood sugar, then that sugar will go on to the unborn child.

Insulin is made by the pancreas, and if the unborn baby is exposed to high levels of sugar, then its own pancreas may develop more insulin secretory cells. In other words, the baby before birth can produce/secrete more insulin. The baby is at a disadvantage before it is even born.

Invariably, the heaviest babies at birth have diabetic mothers. These mothers had higher levels of blood sugar and insulin. This may have been caused by the behavior of the mother to be, or it can be a condition of pregnancy (gestational diabetes)

Pregnant ladies will have their blood glucose levels checked for this reason.

I must state here that some babies are just born big. They are big, happy and healthy, and it has nothing to do with fancy secretory cells or bad behavior by the mother. We are all unique, and some babies are large and perfect in every way.

Insulin, as well as being the fat storing hormone, is also a growth factor and this is why some babies exposed to high levels of insulin are born bigger. For people trying to build muscle they actively create an insulin rich environment as its role as a growth factor will help them build their physique. This is also why it is a challenge to build muscle and get lean at the same time. The most effective way to build muscle involves using insulin and the most effective way of getting lean controls insulin. It is not impossible to do both at the same time, but it takes a person with a confident understanding of how to manipulate insulin to do the job well. The food that we eat can cause a direct insulin response or can overload the liver, and both will trigger lipogenesis the creation of new fat.

We used to believe that fat on our plate led directly to fat of our hips (or in my case back and waist) but now we know that it is the sugar on our plate that paves the most direct route. The carbohydrates that travel to the liver can also end up as stored fat, and these carbs that enter the liver can be repackaged as triglycerides, which then travel in the bloodstream to be stored in adipose tissue/fat cells.

Let me introduce you to Fructose...

We are continually warned about high fructose corn syrup (HFCS), a super sweet additive that is in so many processed foods. Fructose is a highly lipogenic agent; it is easily converted into fat by the liver. Fructose is not metabolized by insulin so does not trigger an insulin response like glucose.

Considering I have just terrorized you about the power of insulin, this might sound like a good thing. Insulin does not remove fructose from the blood; fructose travels straight to the liver. Not a good thing.

The liver does not like an excess of fructose and will convert it into triglycerides. The triglycerides are then sent packing into the bloodstream to be stored as fat.

Fruit sadly gets dragged into the mire right about now. How many times have you heard or said, *"Fruit is all sugar"*?

Yes, fruit does contain simple sugar, but by now you will see that every carbohydrate is sugar. Fruit is both glucose and fructose (single sugars, explained in chapter one). Glucose triggers insulin and the liver converts excess fructose into fat. Fruit, however, is high in fiber and water, also packed with nutrients that the body can use. High Fructose Corn Syrup has none of the benefits of fruit, so it would not be accurate to compare the two.

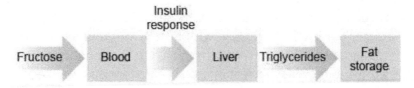

High Fructose Corn Syrup can be found in everything, from bread to hot dogs. In an aggressive retail food industry, a food manufacturer will go to great lengths to make their product taste better than its competition. They do this by adding a sweetness to products that are not even meant to be sweet. If you find yourself preferring one brand to another, check the label, this might be why.

It is unlikely that you are going to gorge on an excess amount of fruit, but you can easily overindulge in high fructose corn syrup without even knowing it.

LIPOPROTEIN LIPASE (LPL)

Lipoprotein lipase (LPL) is an enzyme (a protein that speeds chemical reactions) located in blood vessels. Most LPL is found in adipose tissue (aka fat) and muscle. LPL is responsible for either taking the circulating fat into storage (body fat) or letting active muscle use it as fuel.

LPL activity determines how fat calories are portioned, either they are stored, or they are utilized.

LPL activity may accelerate the rate of fat storage. Changes in body shape and fat patterning can be traced back to increases in LPL activity as we age. Women tend to have more LPL activity in their lower body which causes them to store more fat in their hips and thighs. When LPL is active, it is pulling fat from the blood into the cell, increasing fat storage. Estrogen and testosterone inhibit LPL activity in our mid section. As these hormones decline with age this enzyme ramps up and "hello" middle aged spread. Even if our diet and exercise are unchanged our waistlines tend the thicken. Insulin also plays a part as it stimulates the formation of the LPL enzyme, together they are the power couple of lipogenesis.

LPL activity changes as our sex hormones alter with age but this activity can also be increased with stress and hardcore dieting. Severe or prolonged diets are usually based on the restriction of food, and after a time the body adjusts to make up for the limited intake. Our BMR (basal metabolic rate) is how much energy our body needs in a rested state, and it is expressed as calories. We want our BMR number to be high because we would like to burn a lot of calories, even at rest. The more severe the diet is the more likely the body is to reduce its BMR. If our metabolic rate drops it now takes less energy to do the same amount of work. Essentially chronic dieting can change you from a gas guzzling SUV into a super economical Prius. Generally, in life we seek to be efficient, this is the exception to the rule.

I use a machine that measures basal metabolic rate and without exception, the people who register the lowest are the ones with a history of severe dieting. One lady that visited me was a 26 year old police dog handler who also did CrossFit, spinning and ran half marathons. A terrific lady, 20lb over her goal weight despite eating no more than 1200 calories and zero carbohydrates. To this day she has the lowest metabolic rate I have ever measured, a shocking 830 calories per day.

Compare that to the 70 year old gentleman who came to see me after his heart surgery. As part of his recovery, he had sold his car and walked everywhere. He lived in Santa Monica CA where walking is quicker than driving, so this was a good choice. He said he tried to eat "well" but didn't pay much attention to food. His metabolic rate was 2700 calories.

A 26 year old athlete compared to a 70 year old post heart surgery? By not feeding her body with enough energy to fuel her activity, the policewoman was stuck 20 pounds overweight, half starved and terrified of a day without exercise, whereas the gentleman was active, maintaining his muscle with regular high quality meals and had the metabolism of a (vintage) performance truck.

I can measure a person's metabolic rate, but often there's something else going on, something that becomes apparent when that hard core diet ends. The lipoprotein lipase is in overdrive, all hyped up, ready to grab fat and squirrel it away into storage. It makes total sense, the body has been in a prolonged state of restriction, it adapts by becoming more efficient (BMR drops) and it increases its ability to store fat (LPL activity increases.)

The body is smarter than our dumb actions.

People persevere with the crazy diets, lose the weight, but then what? Few diets give any real follow up plan. Now, these people go back to eating normally, albeit very cautiously. In record speed, all the weight is back (plus some), and it defies math. The amount of food they are eating doesn't equate to the weight gain they are experiencing. Very disheartening as their behavior is better yet they are heavier than when they started. The increased LPL activity coupled with the reduced metabolic capability causes a rapid weight gain, and there is no way around it. The harder you slam your body, the harder it slaps you back.

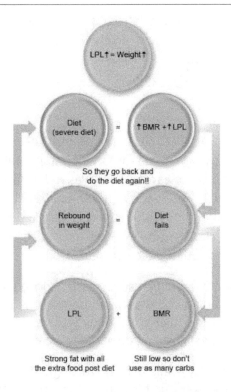

The real sadness is that these people may go back and do the same diet again (and again and again) and a whole new problem arises because yo yo dieters regain much of the weight in their upper body, especially their midsection. They have now accomplished something quite extraordinary; they now have a different body shape.

Lipoprotein lipase is also a regulator when we are stressed. The body can deal with a burst of restricted food intake and it can cope with bouts of stress, but when these situations are ongoing adjustments start to occur. When we suffer from prolonged stress (sleep deprivation, sickness, emotional stress, worry) LPL activity increases. Again, it makes complete sense; in emergency situations, we gather more stores for uncertain times ahead. Think of it like earthquake awareness or a tornado warning; we stock up on everything we might need. Our body is no different.

Lipogenesis is the creation of fat. The hormone insulin transports excess nutrients from the blood into the cell and lipoprotein lipase is the enzyme that controls where and how much fat is stored. Our nutrition, behavior, and stress levels are controllable factors that influence these two players. Declining sex hormones also play a role in body shape and fat distribution.

Time for a happy story.

Lucy, a lady in her late 40s, came to see me; she worked a job that she hated. She had given up her dream of being a ballerina and "sold her soul" for a corporate career. Lucy was quiet, timid and maybe a little sad when I first met her. She didn't exercise, but she did count every calorie she ate and produced a very detailed food journal that spanned months. Her metabolic rate was meager, not much better than the afore mentioned policewoman.

I had another client who did a ballet class and loved it, so I suggested Lucy give it a try. When you work with people one to one, you get a read on someone very quickly. This lady was very self conscious and seemed to have almost given up on herself. She was younger than me!

Five weeks later Lucy walked back through my door a different woman. This firecracker burst into my office, full of chatter. She had gained enough courage to go to the ballet class, she had loved it, but the next time she went along they were about to cancel as the teacher had not shown up. Another student suggested that Lucy lead the class. Lucy said she nearly died; all eyes were on her, she felt pressured and didn't dare refuse.

Long story short: the dance school hired Lucy as a part time instructor. More active and a lot happier, Lucy's metabolic rate had skyrocketed by 400 calories, and she had dropped three inches from her waist.

"Control what you can. Confront what you cannot and always remember how lucky you are to have yourself."

The Maine– American Candy Album

LIPOLYSIS (FAT BREAKDOWN)

Lipolysis is the opposite of lipogenesis. Lipogenesis is the creation of fat and lipolysis is the breakdown of fat.

If your goal is to lose weight your body must be 'in' lipolysis.

You can slap whatever label you want on a diet. You can claim its uniqueness, and how it is going to revolutionize weight loss. But every single diet must do this one thing. It must create an environment of lipolysis: the breakdown of fat. You can't shed stored fat if you don't break it down first.

Lipolysis is a chain reaction involving hormones and enzymes; these reactions release fat from storage sites, and free fatty acids enter the blood. Once in the blood, the fatty acids are available to travel to active tissue to be used as fuel. If they are used for fuel, you lose weight, if they are not used as fuel, they go straight back into storage.

Lipolysis is a chain reaction. A single reaction cannot happen by itself; it depends on the reactions before it. Imagine a line of dominoes, they all fall in sequence, unless you remove one and then the whole chain stops. Your ability to lose weight depends on every step of lipolysis.

I'm not sure why we don't hear about lipolysis more. It always seems to fall on fresh ears when I talk about it, yet we have known about lipolysis for at least half a century

Either the nutrition coach does not know lipolysis, or they may feel it is unnecessary information that takes too long to explain. If the latter is the case, then I feel they are doing their clients a disservice.

I call it my "a ha" moment. As I explain lipolysis I watch my client's expression as the penny drops. In an instant they understand how to lose weight; in an instant they take control back and see where they have been going wrong and how easy it is to fix.

From a business standpoint, I shoot myself in the foot because in no time at all the client doesn't need me. Maybe this is why we don't hear about lipolysis. The weight loss industry relies on repeat business; I prefer to rely on referrals.

We have a bias for storing fat; it takes no special effort on our part to add a few inches here and there. The body has numerous ways to do it and is pretty good at every one of them. Lipogenesis is easy. Lipolysis not so much. Lipolysis is a tightrope that even the most diligent can fall off.

It all starts with epinephrine (aka adrenaline) an excitatory hormone released from the adrenals. Epinephrine is the first domino. Moving on a little farther down the line we have an enzyme called HSL. Hormone Sensitive Lipase (HSL), as the name suggests, is an enzyme that is sensitive to hormones. Once HSL has activated, the fatty acids break free one by one and enter the bloodstream.

Triglycerides is our storage form of fat; three fatty acids, and one glycerol unit. Lipolysis releases these individual units into the bloodstream; they are now available to be used as fuel by active muscles. Lipolysis is the breakdown of fat; it is not fat loss. Lipolysis liberates the fatty acids, but it is diet and exercise that uses those fatty acids as fuel. If the fat in the blood is not used as fuel it travels straight back to the liver where it is repackaged and placed back in storage. This is aptly called a "Futile Cycle."

EXERCISE AND LIPOLYSIS

Muscles love to use fat for fuel. The more muscles we use, the more fat we can burn. Darts and snooker are highly skilled sports, but they don't require a lot of muscle activity, whereas ice skating, running, dancing or cycling are physically demanding and so can burn a lot more fat.

Exercise:

- Increases lipolysis. Exercise has an adrenaline response and adrenaline triggers lipolysis.

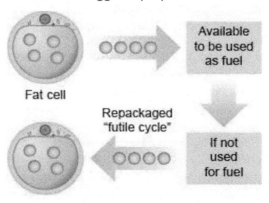

- Increases muscle activity which increases fat burning.

- Increases blood flow. Blood transports release fat to active tissue.

- Trying to lose weight without exercise will be frustrating.

- Choosing an exercise which uses a lot of muscles is advisable.

- Walking works! If you are presently inactive and don't know where to start walk!

HORMONE SENSITIVE LIPASE (HSL)

Remember: Hormone Sensitive Lipase (HSL) is an enzyme that is sensitive to hormones.

Estrogen and testosterone are hormones that decline with age. As these hormones drop, HSL causes lipolysis to slow. We hear the common complaint that losing weight becomes more difficult as we get older. What worked before is no longer enough to get the results we think we deserve. HSL activity is one of the reasons why HSL is suppressed, lipolysis slows, and stored fat is broken down at a slower rate.

Sound familiar?

- Sex hormones decline, and fat breakdown slows.

- Sex hormones decline and LPL activity increases.

- Fat breakdown slows and fat storage increases.

- A cruel (double) twist of fate.

INSULIN AND HSL

You may be familiar with the term "You're either pregnant, or you're not." It is used to express how absolute a situation is.

You are either in lipolysis or you are not.

"The most sensitive endpoint that INSULIN has is its ability to shut down lipolysis."

For some of you, this one sentence will be the most powerful thing you will ever hear. That one sentence will forever change the way you eat.

A few pages back you read that when there is too much sugar (carbohydrates) in the blood, the hormone insulin is over released. Insulin is a storage facilitator and takes that sugar into fat storage.

Insulin "insulates" and is our fat storage hormone.

You cannot be in two environments at the same time. You cannot be hot and cold at the same time, or tired and energetic simultaneously. In the same way, you can't be breaking fat down if you are busy storing it. It would make no sense.

As we know, storing fat is lipogenesis and breaking fat down is lipolysis; they cannot occur at the same time, and the way this is prevented is by insulin deactivating HSL. If there is no HSL activation, lipolysis stops, fat breakdown stops, weight loss stops.

INSULIN, A HORMONE

HSL, an enzyme sensitive to hormones

One cancels the other out.

Going back to that killer conclusion, "The most sensitive endpoint that insulin has, is its ability to shut down lipolysis." The first time I heard this I was listening to a Berkley Clinical Nutrition Lecture. I was in Golds Gym Venice CA, running on the treadmill and listening to the lecture on my iPod (yes, that long ago). I had a slew of nutrition certifications, I lived in the fitness capital of the world, had been on the Olympia stage, and this was my first time hearing this.

It changed everything for me, and I hope it does the same for you.

Moreover, be clear: if your carbohydrate intake causes elevated blood sugar, then you will shut down lipolysis: you will not slow it down, it will stop, fat breakdown will stop. Lipolysis will not start up again until insulin and blood sugar are under control.

Here's a thought; what if every meal a person ate shut down lipolysis for a few hours? If they ate three meals and some snacks would they ever even be in lipolysis?

This explains why gyms are full of people that never change. It is the reason recreational runners gain weight and why going vegetarian might cause the scale to go up not down.

INSULIN = *halts* HSL = *halts* LIPOLYSIS

Carbohydrates trigger insulin.

Protein has a slight insulin response.

Fat has no insulin response.

Lipolysis is halted by your carbohydrate intake and/or the size of your meal.

If carbohydrates trigger insulin and insulin shuts down lipolysis, we should go zero carbs and be skinny, right?

There would be more truth in that idea if only it were all so simple. However, it is true that controlling blood sugar by controlling carbohydrate intake is essential for weight loss.

STUBBORN FAT

We all have our problem areas. It might be your thighs or your back, it might be the love handles hanging over your jeans or the pouch right below your belly button. Wherever it is, it drives you mad. It is true that some areas metabolize fat at a slower rate and seem resistant to diet and exercise. How many women have I seen with lean upper bodies and hips that don't match? How many men sport a six pack and a roll under each shoulder blade?

Stubborn fat and fat patterning can be explained by recognizing your body type. As I say, I see myself as a mesomorph/androgenic. My legs can stay lean, but I won't wear a backless dress. When I reduce my bodyfat that back fat will hold on for dear life and be the last to go.

Identifying with your body type will help with the frustration, but stubborn fat can have other causes. Let's start with the those you can fix.

Nutrition is not just about losing weight, and losing weight is not just about nutrition. An unhealthy diet will burden the liver, which has to deal with everything we throw at it; it has to break down alcohol, medication, environmental toxins and so the list of aggressors goes on. If you are bombarding the liver, it can become a toxic place. High carbohydrate sugary foods combined with pills, booze, and too little exercise will make it more difficult for us to break down body fat. A poor diet low in B vitamins, chromium, zinc, protein and omega 3 fatty acids will affect your fat burning ability, no doubt about it.

Moving towards less processed foods (easier for the liver to handle), staying away from foods that you are allergic or intolerant to (digestive stress), limiting alcohol, controlling insulin, managing stress and making exercise a priority, are all ways you can improve your ability to burn fat.

Cruciferous vegetables like broccoli, bok choy, Brussels sprouts, cauliflower, cabbage and similar vegetables are good for detoxifying the liver. They contain Inol 3 Carbinol which you can find in supplement form as DIM (diindolylmethane). Milk thistle and dandelion root are also excellent for cleansing the liver, as well as SAM (adenosylmethionine) which, along with its other uses, is a popular liver supplement.

You are only as good as your body's ability to digest and absorb what you consume.

Second generation fat is more stubborn than the first. It gets harder to lose weight the second, third, fourth time around. Yo yo dieting will cause more weight gain in the upper body and arms, and that fat will become harder and harder to lose.

INSULIN RESISTANCE (IR)

High carbohydrate diets with little exercise create an environment of high blood sugar and too much sugar in the blood triggers too much insulin. This behavior is the course towards insulin resistance.

Unbeknownst to the host, cells stop responding to insulin. Insulin is a hormone, hormones are messengers, and cells stop listening to the message. Insulin tries to get sugar out of the blood but if the cells don't listen then the sugar (and the insulin) stay in the blood and levels get dangerously high.

By now you know what this means. High blood sugar and high insulin will shut down lipolysis. Fat is not going anywhere and could be considered 'stubborn,' but this is not true.

Get rid of the sugar, watch your carbs, relax more, get good sleep. Laugh every day, drink less of the fun stuff, drink more of the good stuff, don't pop pills, do move, stretch and sweat. Watch that fat fall off hopefully.

If you are doing all the right things and that fat is still the friend that won't leave, then the term 'stubborn fat' may apply.

There is an explanation.

In lipolysis, the chain of reactions starts with epinephrine (adrenaline). We have focused on Hormone Sensitive Lipase (HSL) and its crucial role in lipolysis, but before we even get to HSL epinephrine has to bind with the receptors of the fat cell.

Hormones are just messengers; they do not do anything by themselves; they travel around the body and bind to their matching receptors. Again, think of that lock and key. Alone neither do anything but put the right key in the right lock and doors open. In the same way, hormones attach to their specific receptors, the message is relayed, and things start to happen.

Estrogen can only attach itself to estrogen receptors. Insulin connects with cells that have insulin receptors, and epinephrine (the first step in lipolysis) has to bind to its own unique receptor sites.

There are two types of receptors. Alpha (types 1 and 2) and Beta (types 1, 2 and 3).

The body always seeks balance, and to create balance we need regulators. You regulate the temperature of your home by using heat and AC. You regulate the speed of your car by using the accelerator and the brake.

Cells have Alpha and Beta receptors which work very much like an accelerator or a brake. These two types of receptors can speed up a reaction or slow it down. Lipolysis is a reaction, and when epinephrine binds to the receptors on the fat cell, it can go either way. Activation of Alpha 1 and Beta receptors will allow for the breakdown of fat, while activation of Alpha 2 is anti lipolytic and it will slow fat breakdown. If there are more Alpha 2 receptors, then they will dominate, and fat breakdown will be blunted. When we have an area of stubborn fat, it may be that there are more Alpha 2 receptors.

Your foot is the hormone but what your foot does depends on which pedal you hit.

Muscle cells have Alpha and Beta receptors; the latter stimulate protein synthesis and help in muscle building. A lack of Beta receptors may be a limiting factor for a hard gainer.

Women struggle with lower body weight to the point where there is a dramatic difference between their upper bodies and their butt, hips and thighs. Hormones, LPL activity, and Alpha receptor activation may be an explanation.

Competitive pool players and golfers may take beta blockers so that they are calm and can concentrate on their game. Beta receptors are the accelerators, they increase heart rate. In a sport that demands accuracy, it does not help if your heart is racing and this is where beta blockers can prove useful.

Beta blockers are banned, in competitive sports because of the unfair advantage they can give, but there is no "anti doping committee" in the weight loss world. There have been many attempts to block the Alpha 2 receptors or specifically stimulate the Beta.

A few decades ago, ephedra was a very popular weight loss and performance supplement. It was like slamming your foot on the accelerator, giving yourself a crazy amount of short lived energy. Spin classes were full of people hopped up on this over the counter supplement. Truck drivers could drive all night and girls got bikini ready in record time due to ephedra and its synthetic partner ephedrine HCL.

Ephedra was banned and there are two sides to that story like every story. Human nature does push up towards the "more is better" mentality, and there was no doubt an unsafe mass abuse of this product. Lipolysis starts with ephedrine, and ephedra products boosted that first step in fat breakdown. People were taking the process into their own hands. BUT it did not work for everyone.

Ladies took ephedrine to get rid of that stubborn body fat, but because those parts of their body were dominant in Alpha 2 receptors, it proved ineffective. The mistake was then to take more and more ephedra, torsos got shredded, and butts continued to jiggle.

While Alpha 2 receptors were slamming on the brakes in the stubborn fat, the gas pedal was being slammed everywhere else, and you know what happens to an engine when you rev the gas too hard for too long...

Ephedra is "Non Specific," and its success as a fat burner is dependent on the ratio of Alpha and Beta receptors. Chronic use of ephedra during calorie restriction can have an anabolic effect, and it can increase levels of the thyroid hormone T3.

I witnessed these many times back in the 90's. Due to the anabolic effect ladies could get hard muscular upper bodies and a little fuzzy facial hair. I recall one lady losing 30% in body fat while dropping only a few pounds from her glutes and thighs. She was burnt out within a year of competing and fell into a major depression. Depression is an unavoidable pitfall after stimulant abuse.

Alpha and Beta receptors allow for balance.

Some people with access turned to Clenbuterol (popular with racehorses) which is "Beta Specific." If you specifically hit the Beta receptors you speed everything up. This was a game changer, people gained muscle and lost body fat which, in theory, is great but no action works in isolation. A Beta specific drug will hit every beta receptor, including those in the heart and the lungs.

If you keep revving an engine, it will blow.

There have been natural attempts to swing the balance in favor of lipolysis. Some herbal remedies like Yohimbine bark are "Alpha Antagonists" used to inhibit the Alpha 2 receptors.

I wish I could recommend a solution to stubborn fat, but I cannot. Receptors create balance, and I am never going to suggest messing with that. What I can offer up is one priceless nugget of information.

Insulin makes the Alpha 2 receptors more sensitive.

At the end of the day, it all comes back to nutrition.

GENERATION FAT

We have billions of fat cells, and each cell holds a droplet of fat. That fat (aka lipid) takes up about 85% of the cell's volume, while the other 15% is the cell's nucleus (the message center) and cytoplasm (usually water, salt, and protein). When we lose weight, we do not lose fat cells; rather we reduce the volume of each cell. A balloon half filled with water weighs less than a balloon filled with water.

If you have four times more fat cells than your friend and you both have fat cells that are 85% lipid, then you are going to be much larger and much heavier than that pal of yours. To get to be the same weight you're going to have to drastically reduce the volume of each cell and here lies the frustration of weight loss and achieving long lasting results.

The role of homeostasis is to bring about balance. Fat cells strive to return to their former volume. The person that swears their eating did not warrant their rebound in weight. They may well be telling the truth.

There are thought to be three times in our life when we can increase the number of fat cells in our body; the third trimester of pregnancy (before we are born), our first year of life and also during puberty.

We had no control over what our mothers ate or fed to us before or after our birth, and body composition isn't a real priority during puberty.

Today the challenge for children is fast food, soda, and candy on every corner, on every shelf and on every commercial. Children are not as active, and there is more screen time than playtime. Large children are becoming the norm.

The sadness here is that without even knowing it, children and their parents are setting the stage for adulthood. Children go through so many physical changes as they barrel towards adulthood. We call it 'puppy fat' and often that's all it is. The podgy nine year old girl that transforms into a svelte 14 year old. The 11 year old boy that grows taller than his mom in one school year.

And then there's that heavy kid that doesn't lose the weight.

The depressing fact is that 75% of obese children become obese adults and these kids are adding new fat cells at twice the rate of their lean counterparts. Of normal weight children, only 10% will become obese adults.

Obesity which is said to be 25 40% hereditary; two obese adults have a child, and there is an 80 90% chance that their child will also be obese. Two normal weight people have a child, and there is only a 10 15% chance their child will be obese. One obese parent brings the odds to 40 50%.

Please don't fixate on these percentages; it's doubtful that they are carved in stone, and I merely use them to illustrate how our body composition has a firm hold on us before we even choose to make it a priority.

The changing shape and size of society is going to cripple the health of future generations, and the cost will be astronomical. I like to think that I am full of good advice, but I am at a loss as to how to reverse it all. Heavy kids make for heavy adults, and heavy adults make for heavy kids. The mathematical certainty of it all is quite daunting and makes me grateful for being a child of the 70's.

FAT HAS A MIND OF ITS OWN

We used to think that fat was just unsightly rolls of 'future' fuel. Stores of potential energy that we probably would never need.

That's what we used to think. We now know that fat is an active organ that secretes dozens of hormones and gives out its own chemical messages. In fact, fat is quite the chatterbox!

Hormones like leptin and adiponectin listen to fat. Leptin, discovered in 1994, is a protein that is made in fat cells and travels in the blood to tell your brain how much energy you have in storage. If you start to lose too much fat leptin levels drop and at some point, your brain gets concerned enough that it increases your appetite to encourage you to eat more. You eat more, gain some weight and leptin levels return to normal. Leptin and your brain don't care that you want a six pack.

Have you noticed how much food a hardcore dieter can eat when they have a cheat meal? Have you ever noticed how your appetite is greater after every diet? Have you ever come across that person that doesn't have much of an appetite? I bet they don't diet.

Adiponectin is another protein discovered in the 1990's. Adiponectin is linked to insulin and insulin sensitivity. Remember, insulin is the hormone that controls the sugar (carbohydrates) in our blood. Insulin transports nutrients into cells (including fat cells), and we want to be sensitive.

If we are insulin sensitive, then insulin can effectively and efficiently control the sugar in our blood. If we are resistant to insulin, the pancreas must release more and more of this powerful hormone for it to do its job.

Obese people have less adiponectin and are more resistant to insulin. Lean people have more adiponectin and tend to be sensitive to insulin. Low adiponectin levels are a marker for inflammation, and inflammation is a trigger for diabetes and heart disease.

There are more than 80 different proteins made by fat cells. In fact There are more than 80 different proteins made by fat cells, we don't know too much about them all yet, but you can bet they hold the answer as to why excess fat is linked to our most serious health conditions.

Obese people, on average, die ten years earlier than those that are of normal weight and the years that they live are often plagued by diabetes, cancers and heart disease.

Recalling the types of fat, we can see dangerous patterns, evidenced in a difference between the sexes. Visceral fat is the abdominal fat that looks like a pot belly, and it is the most dangerous fat to carry. As we age we gain less subcutaneous fat (the fat underneath the skin) and more fat collects as visceral fat around the midsection. Women carry more fat than men but have less fat related health issues. It is thought that this is because women have more subcutaneous fat and less visceral fat than men. This sneaky visceral fat is that stuff that collects around our internal organs and is associated with high blood pressure, insulin resistance, low HDL (good cholesterol), high LDL (bad cholesterol), increased risk of diabetes and cardiovascular disease.

We live with a body that is way smarter than our thoughts and desires. Homeostasis means to find a balance that is what our body seeks, and it has a great many ways to achieve it. For every action, there is a reaction, and no event ever occurs in isolation. When it comes to losing weight, it is too easy and far too simplistic to rely on that adage "Eat Less, Move More". Once you pass 40, it is unlikely to be that straightforward. Nuance and careful understanding come into play.

CHAPTER THREE: HOW TO LOSE WEIGHT & WHY WE DON'T

The Minnesota Semi Starvation Study, discussed in the introduction, was not embarked upon to help us drop a pant size and yet 60 years on we can learn so much from the experiences of those 36 men.

Recap:

36 men of healthy mind and body spent three months eating normally. This was followed by six months of food restriction; 1500 calories per day. The study concluded with a three month refeed.

- On average the men lost 25% of their body weight in the six months of restriction.

- The men experienced dramatic changes which in many cases lasted well into the rehabilitation phase.

- The men's interest in food increased to the point of obsession.

- The men became ritualistic with their eating; this behavior spilled into other areas of their lives.

- They dreamt about food, collected photographs of food, became interested in nutrition and found enjoyment in watching others eat.

- Some men ate secretly, collecting food paraphernalia like plates and silverware. They would hoard these items, and they would begin to hoard in general.

- The men drank a lot of coffee, chewed a lot of gum and would spend money on meaningless purchases, something that they had never done before the six months of food restriction.

- Not surprisingly, all the men experienced hunger. Some did okay, and others binged, eating vast amounts of food.

Enormous self loathing followed.

- The men became withdrawn, they lost any sense of humor and lost interest in their relationships and sex.

- Most of the men lost control of their appetite, even following the three month refeed/rehabilitation phase. Men ate 10,000 calories and were still hungry.

- The volunteers were both physically and mentally healthy and yet at least 20% of them suffered emotional distress and said they could not function normally. Many of them experienced extreme depression and some had intense mood swings.

- Symptoms included irritability, anger, negativity, argumentativeness, depression, nail biting, smoking and self neglect around personal hygiene.

Does any of this sound familiar?

If you haven't experienced any of these behaviors, you have probably witnessed them.

- These men had a hard time focusing. They became sensitive to light and cold and suffered intestinal discomfort.

- Their metabolic rate dropped by 40% and they became weak.

I competed for 13 years, and I can attest to experiencing at least half of what these men put themselves through.

Looking at highlights on social media, not much has changed. I watch as fitness competitors isolate themselves with hoodies and headphones, unable to deal with anything other than meal prep and their next workout.

The word 'bloat' abounds as a conjunction in every other sentence. I have watched the weight rebound, and I know many of these people will be desperately unhappy.

The real sadness is that in the fitness world this is expected and accepted. It is the norm. Before the body has had the chance to recover it is on the next diet.

The Minnesota starvation study was 36 healthy men without a history of food restriction. I had done at least 35 diets before the age of 30. It took my body two years to find its peace.

Weight loss is not impossible, but this 70 year old study reminds us that to achieve lasting results we must work with our body and not against it. In short, we come back to that guiding gem: *"The body is way smarter than our dumb actions."*

All industries change over time. For example, the medical industry, which is closely associated with nutrition, health, and weight loss, continually advances as more becomes known about the complexities of biology. Virus discoveries changed how surgeries are performed. Until they were understood – understood to even exist – the risk of infection had not been appreciated, or even acknowledged. Personal cleanliness and sterile conditions were then demanded, lives were saved, and cures were found. The era of a hot blade and whiskey ended with the discovery of the virus.

What we know about weight loss has dramatically changed over the last 40 years. Calories used to be all we knew, and diets were based on restricting them. Eating less and moving more is still great advice for most people, especially in this sedentary age, but when restriction and expenditure, are taken too far, these same tools will be used against us.

Thankfully we know so much more about what influences body composition. The discussion has grown quite complex and yet is even more fascinating. We have come so far that my client presentations may not even include the word "calorie".

FOOD AND FAT

This is ground which we have covered but, as it is central to this book, let's return to it from a slightly different direction; how we might think daily about what is going on in our bodies when we eat.

The carbohydrates that we eat appear in the blood as single units of sugar. We call this "blood glucose" or "blood sugar".

If blood sugar is too high, insulin is over released, and insulin traps stored fat in its cell. To lose weight we need to release fat from its storage site. Insulin stops this from happening.

Every meal you eat will dictate your ability to use fat stores for fuel.

Too many nutrients in the blood is not a good thing, and too many carbohydrates are the lightning rod for various health conditions and diseases.

When we have too many carbohydrates/glucose in the blood we create an environment called "high blood sugar." In a healthy person, this is created by:

- Eating too many carbohydrates in one sitting.

- Eating meals too close together

- Eating a meal that is too large.

One or more of these three factors will lead to elevated blood sugar, and the body does not like that.

The assumption was that if you restricted energy intake and increased energy expenditure then you would lose weight. The idea was that stored body fat would fill any deficit created. A straightforward and logical approach that was easy to grasp and made sense to many people. It is true, but only as far as it goes, and for some people that will not be far enough.

Understanding comes before belief. We thought we understood weight loss and so we believed in this approach and this belief became so deep rooted that it is still tough for people to let go of.

The fragile theory hinges on the idea that the body uses fuel and when there isn't enough fuel it will burn fat. However, stored fat is 'future' energy, and our bodies are not that excited to get rid of it, especially in uncertain times. Furthermore, the body does have options.

We have a strong bias for being fat. It was once considered a thing of beauty. In 1908 a female stone figure known as the Venus of Willendorf was discovered. She was a big girl, and she dates from way back, around 25,000 B.C. In such harsh times, (14,000 years before the end of the cycle of Ice Ages), being obese was highly desirable. It was even celebrated by sculpting obese figures who would be catcalled of the catwalk.

Consider our bodies' bias for being fat and staying fat. Lack of sleep, stress, excess food, medications, hormones; all can facilitate the body slipping into its natural, comfortable, fat storage mode. In cruel contrast, the body offers only one skinny little pathway to get rid of our fat reserves. Take even one step off the path and fat breakdown stops.

FUEL

On the plus side, the body, from the neck down, loves to use fat for fuel, it has a great affinity for burning fat for fuel, it is set up to burn fat for fuel. However, it doesn't NEED to use fat for fuel.

The body is happy to use blood glucose for fuel. Indeed, if there is sugar to be had, it will use that before it even considers using our stored body fat.

The body can use fuel stored in the liver (glycogen), it can use fuel stored in the muscle (glycogen) and, at a pinch, it will break down lean muscle tissue.

From the neck down the body loves to use fat for fuel (dietary and body fat) but it does have other options.

From the neck up, the brain and nervous system only allow for minor utilization of fatty acids. Fatty acids can be oxidized to provide fuel for the heart, lungs, kidneys and muscles but the brain doesn't oxidize these acids very well. This could be because they cross the blood brain barrier too slowly, or it may be because there is not enough enzyme activity to degrade the fatty acids upon arrival. The fuel of choice is, therefore, glucose, which primarily comes from the carbohydrates you consume.

Oxidation is the moving of electrons. A substance that gives away electrons is "oxidized". The obvious example of oxidization is when iron reacts to oxygen; it is oxidized and forms rust. Fatty acid oxidation refers to the fatty acids being broken down and energy being released. The brain does not do this well.

Blood sugar is the best available fuel for the brain and nervous system. However, note that the brain does not limit itself to one source of fuel; if that were the case, we would have been extinct thousands of years ago.

The Ketogenic Diet has been around for decades and in recent years has gained renewed popularity, and for good reason. Through nutrition, we can create an environment that allows ketones to be produced and used as a very efficient form of energy for every cell in the body and brain.

Ketones come from fat and, at first, this made people over the age of 40 pretty uncomfortable.

I would do the Ketogenic Diet an injustice if I tried to fully explain it in a few paragraphs, but it would be remiss to exclude a brief explanation of how ketosis works and why it has a die hard fan base.

To understand ketosis is to illustrate, yet again, the body's wondrous ability to adapt to circumstance.

The carbohydrates we eat make sugar/glucose/glycogen the most abundant fuel, but what if you take those carbs away for a prolonged period? At first, you will use your stored carbohydrates; we have some in the liver and in the muscle (glycogen), and maybe we have a few hundred calories floating around in the blood. What happens when that's all gone?

If we're not eating any carbohydrates and we don't have any stored then we move to plan B: the body, when pushed, can convert protein into a source of glucose. Now that is amazing. It's called "gluconeogenesis" aka "new glucose."

The ketogenic diet removes carbohydrates, limits protein and instead uses a lot of quality fats. Stored carbohydrates are gone, and gluconeogenesis does not provide enough glucose. It is then that the magic happens; fat is taken to the liver and converted into ketones. Ketones run freely around the body providing an abundance of energy for every cell including the brain cells.

Fat (dietary and body fat) can now become the primary fuel. People who have struggled to lose weight now drop it with ease, pain vanishes, health conditions improve. It's a game changer for so many people.

Achieving ketosis and becoming "keto adapted" is not merely eating a low carb diet and, although I am a big fan of keto, hope by now you get the often complex picture and therefore understand that the Ketogenic Diet won't work for everyone.

There are 16 recognized personality types, some love structure, some thrive on spontaneity, some work best with repetition and others variety. We are in different life stages with different lifestyles and different obligations. One diet does not fit all. Leaving physiological factors aside, the success of any diet is contingent upon what our individual personality is likely to comply with.

THE BRAIN AND BLOOD SUGAR

When the brain and the nervous system has blood sugar for fuel, all is well in the world. The nervous system communicates with every other system in the body respiratory, muscular, digestive, endocrine and circulatory. If the nervous system is tweaked because it doesn't have enough fuel, it's not going to send out a positive message of cheer.

How well do you communicate when you're hungry?

This shows up as cravings, irritability, moodiness, lack of focus, dizziness and sometimes headaches. When we go too long without eating there is no fuel in our blood, there is no fuel to cross the blood brain barrier; there is no fuel going to the brain. The initial symptoms are hunger and cravings.

In reality, the body isn't going to rely on us eating; it does have the ability to release stored carbohydrates (glycogen) when dietary fuel is low. To say "no fuel" is available is dramatic of me, although when you haven't eaten for a while, this is how it feels and that is the signal the brain will send out

When blood sugar is low we don't crave chicken breast. We crave sugar, we crave something sweet, we crave the very thing the brain and nervous system prefer to feed on; we crave blood sugar.

Our body can use fat for fuel. However, fat remains trapped in storage if there are too many carbohydrates in the blood. Elevated blood sugar triggers our storage hormone, insulin, which locks fat in the cells.

Carbohydrates in the blood will always be the primary fuel of choice. To lose body fat, we must release fat from storage and we can only do this by controlling our carbohydrate intake.

The answer would seem simple. Eliminate carbohydrates and fat will be used for fuel. Many of you will have tried this approach already with varying degrees of success. Remembering that the brain feeds primarily on glucose, a drastic drop in carbohydrates may lead to bad behavior. The classic example is when you feel like you were so good all day, but as soon as you got home, you dropped to your knees and ate everything in the refrigerator.

The problem here is that people identify with their own behavior. They will say they are binge eaters or sugar addicts. In truth, their food choices continually create a state of unstable blood sugar. It's not them, there is no personal failing or flaw but that belief, about themselves, can be the one thing that holds them back.

Reducing carbohydrates can be very uncomfortable, though usually only at first.

The brain requires 5.6mg of glucose per 100 grams of brain tissue per minute about 120 grams of glucose per day. The brain prefers a continuous supply of glucose, so we can simplify the math one step further and say the brain requires 5 grams per hour.

20 grams of most carbohydrates is the size of a deck of cards,

including rice, potato, bread and pasta.

Carbohydrates are inexpensive compared to protein, so most meals are carb dense. Consider the carbohydrate serving size we are accustomed to (and expect). Herein lies the problem.

We do not need to eat a lot of carbohydrates to keep the brain happy, and we do not have to eliminate carbohydrates to lose weight.

Very Low Calorie Diets (VLCD) that are high in carbohydrates will have limited results and are torturous to follow. The inclusion of carbohydrates will trigger an insulin response, and although insulin needs an excess of nutrients to store fat, even the limited intake will allow insulin to maintain body fat levels. Any progress will be tediously slow, muscle will be wasted, metabolisms will be crushed and willpower exhausted. Painful and so unnecessary: weight will be regained, and blame will be assigned to oneself.

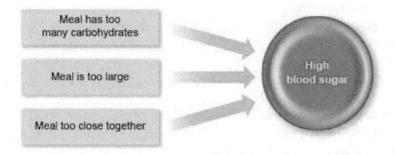

A 1200 calorie diet that is 45 65% carbohydrates (as suggested by the Mayo Clinic) equals 135 195 grams of carbohydrates per day. Most people will be very hungry on 1200 calories a day so long term compliance is unlikely.

A diet of 1800 calories a day with 25 35% carbohydrates equals 113 158 grams of carbohydrates a day.

The higher calories per day diet will still provide the brain what it needs while allowing for lower blood sugar, the release of stored fat and an intake that is metabolically protective and keeps you from chewing your arm off.

The upshot is hard to miss. Firstly, compliance is key to success. And secondly, counting calories does not guarantee results.

A training client of mine was trying to lose weight. I checked his blood sugar and it was dangerously high. We drastically changed his diet and I asked him to test his blood sugar several times a day. Over two weeks we brought his blood glucose down from over 400 (milligrams of glucose per deciliter of blood) to 180 ml/dl.

(In the UK and Canada, the number is expressed as millimoles per liter mmol/l. To convert to ml/dl multiply by 18.)

My guy had made drastic nutritional changes and expected just as dramatic results, but he only lost a couple of pounds in those first few weeks. His blood sugar had dropped from a level that scared the heck out of me to a number that was closing in on normal, but there was still too much sugar in his blood and fat remained trapped.

It was incredibly frustrating for my client to reap such paltry reward from his fine efforts, but once I explained what was happening he understood that it was going to take more than a few weeks of good eating to turn around decades of bad behavior. My client persevered; he tested his own blood sugar several times a day, and that proved to be a motivating force. Eventually, the pounds started to come off.

Normal blood glucose would be a morning reading of under 100 ml/dl and no higher than 140 ml/dl two hours after eating. The power of testing blood sugar is that eating behavior becomes real. We can talk carbohydrates and count grams, but that blood test is the best mode of compliance bar none. A blood glucose meter is sold as a diabetic tool, but I would argue that if we got used to testing our own blood sugar we would avoid type 2 diabetes in the first place.

I will ask new clients to eat as usual for a few days and to test their blood sugar 30 minutes after each meal. This alone can change eating behavior. If those chicken fajitas resulted in a reading above 200, there is a good chance you won't order that meal again. If that green drink you have for lunch pushed you into the high 180's (true story) you will likely make a different choice.

When you give people good information they can relate to, they make better choices all by themselves, with natural ease.

Based on my own observations, I suggest keeping blood glucose under 120 ml/dl if the goal is weight loss. If we use a low carbohydrate, higher fat diet then I may ask to keep the reading sub 100.

All diets have one thing in common; they create an environment to lower blood sugar. They may slap a different label on the diet to emphasize uniqueness but they all lower blood glucose levels to allow stored fat to be released.

Paleo, Atkins, Warrior, Jenny Craig, Weight Watchers or South Beach. They use their methods to lower blood glucose, and they all have their strengths. South Beach and Paleo work for the health conscious, a Warrior diet attracts a certain personality type. Even the dinosaurs of the industry use social accountability and support which can be a big help.

This is not a diet book because I cannot hang my hat on any one diet.

Controlling blood sugar in a way that allows for ease of long term compliance determines success. It doesn't sound as sexy as "Warrior" but that's the bottom line.

Nutrition should fit into your lifestyle, not your lifestyle into nutrition.

HORMONES

Let's consider hormones in terms of daily lifestyle. Hormones are chemical messengers that travel through our body triggering other events to happen.

Think of hormones like emails. Emails are sent out into the abyss, and yet they only reach the person that they are addressed to. When opened, they trigger events. Hormones travel in our blood yet only attach to their specific receptor sites. Testosterone can only attach to testosterone receptors. Cortisol, a stress hormone, can only attach to cortisol receptors, insulin can only attach to insulin receptors, and so on.

Hormones are released from glands, they attach to receptors, and this stirs events within the body. Consequently, our hormonal environment governs our body composition, our energy and how we age.

If your hormones are out of balance you can cut calories and you can exercise until your feet bleed and you may not lose a single pound. Ladies in menopause can attest to this.

Hormones can be fat soluble. These fat soluble hormones are made on demand and cannot be stored. Thyroid, aldosterone, vitamin D, progesterone, testosterone, estrogen and cortisol are fat soluble hormones. Water soluble hormones can be stored. Adrenaline, insulin, glucagon and growth hormone are water soluble hormones.

Too much or too little of a hormone is a diseased state, and hormone effectiveness depends on hormone receptors. Too much of the stress hormone cortisol can cause Cushing's syndrome, and too little cortisol may lead to Addison's Disease. Our hormone balance is a delicate and never ending juggle. The interplay between hormones and health – specifically with regard to weight and well being – becomes more manageable once we are aware of it.

When the conversation is weight loss the hormone we are talking about first is insulin.

INSULIN AND INSULIN RESISTANCE

Insulin was discovered in 1921 and, as previously mentioned, it was used as a treatment for anorexics in the 1930s who did indeed gain weight. The power of this hormone was clearly considerable, and it was applied to other mental disorders, such as depression. (In the movie A Beautiful Mind with Russell Crowe you may recall how they used insulin in shock therapy, and all the patients gained weight.) However, it was not until the 1960's that we were able to measure insulin.

Fat tissue is the most sensitive to insulin and insulin is a driving force for appetite and hunger, so it is for good reason that insulin has been branded 'the fat hormone.' However, it might be more helpful to think of it as our 'storage hormone.' With excess nutrients, insulin will store fat, which we don't like, but insulin also drives amino acids into muscle cells to allow for muscle growth, which we do like.

Poor diet, lack of exercise or advanced age can cause 'insulin resistance' meaning the storage system stops working. It is always the muscle tissue that becomes resistant first. When the insulin receptors on muscle cells fail to function, even more nutrients go into fat storage. If fat cell receptors fail, then insulin cannot take nutrients there either.

Insulin Resistance is one of those terms we hear a lot as if we're expected to know what it means, but it is rarely explained. Insulin has receptors on muscle, fat and liver cells. The main nutrient that triggers insulin is carbohydrates although the amino acids of protein do also elicit a milder insulin response. Leucine is an amino acid and is the most favored amino acids for muscle growth. Leucine triggers insulin but not to the extent of carbohydrates.

Consider someone eating a lot of carbohydrates (potatoes, sugar, cereal, bread, candy, pasta, etc.); they constantly have elevated blood sugar and their pancreas is constantly churning out insulin to cope. The receptors are inundated by insulin and start to fail. Muscle cells become resistant which forces more nutrients into fat cells, hence type 2 diabetics get fat at first.

If the situation continues a type 2 diabetic may become very thin. If fat cells become resistant nutrients have nowhere to go, so they stay in the blood. The diabetic now has high blood levels of both insulin and sugar. Organs, tissue, limbs and sight may now be affected. If this dire situation in left to fester, the majority of type 2 diabetics will die from cardiovascular episodes such as a heart attack or strokes.

Imagine moving into a house next to a rail track. At first, when a train goes past the noise drives you crazy. You're not going to be able to hold a conversation and the trains are going to wake you up. Over time you grow accustomed to the noise, and the trains barely disrupt. When you are continually exposed to something you become acclimatized to it; you no longer respond to it, you become "resistant" to it.

Eating too much sugar with too little exercise will make you fat. Fat people are less likely to exercise because that extra weight is hard to move. This does not mean that every person with a lot of body fat is diabetic and unfit. It is unkind to make this assumption. However, it would be nonsense to deny that resistance to exercise is a bedfellow or resistance to insulin.

Of course, assumptions are dodgy per se with health and food. For another classic example; to merely presume a normal weight person must be healthy is folly. Our choices and behavior are the true indicators of our health. Ectomorphs do not get a health pass just because of their weight.

We have all experienced a food coma. We eat too much food and feel extremely tired afterward. The food we ate spiked our blood sugar and the resulting insulin carried the nutrients out of the blood and into muscle (maybe) and into fat. Now the nutrients are out of the blood we are left with low blood sugar, so exhaustion sets in.

Ironically high blood sugar always leads to low blood sugar; it causes that energy crash which leads to cravings and hunger. Remember from the earlier section, 'Insulin and LPL', this sudden drop in energy after a meal leading to hunger is just insulin doing its thing. And in daily terms, it's manageable so long as you know that is all that's going on and you don't succumb to cravings and pig out after an already large meal.

Doubly ironic and very annoying are the products that claim to give you energy. Energy bars and drinks are full of sugar and will inevitably make you crash. If you need a short burst of energy, they may be of some use, but if you need to make it through the day, you better buy a case. And that brings us back to the quiet, daily nurturing of insulin resistance.

MUSCLE FUEL & "CARBING UP"

If you're involved in endurance sports you may have been told to "carb up" for an event. The theory runs that if you eat a lot of carbohydrates, they will be transported into your muscle to fuel your big day. Let me tell you from experience, there are so many things that can go wrong here. It took me my first ten years of competing to get this exactly right, so it is very VERY doubtful that an online coach or social media 'guru' will nail it for you. Unless you're working with someone that really knows how to manipulate your nutrient intake, you're more likely to get it wrong than right. Too many carbohydrates at the wrong time will make you tired and sluggish and fat.

By now you know the basics but note the wording. Insulin can take carbohydrates into muscle. Muscle stores carbohydrates as glycogen. Glycogen will fuel that muscle's activity.

There are a couple of keywords to heed there. Insulin CAN take nutrients into muscle but sometimes it CAN'T. Glycogen will fuel THAT muscle's activity it will not fuel ANOTHER muscle's activity.

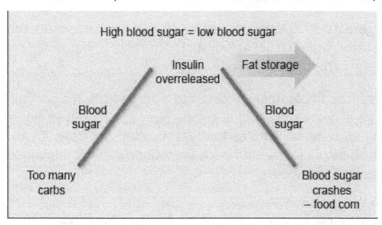

To see this full picture, which is perfectly comprehensible and very important, keep the terminology in mind. Carbohydrates are on your plate. Carbohydrates in your blood are called blood sugar or blood glucose. Carbohydrates in your muscle (or liver) are referred to as glycogen.

If we freeze water, we call it ice, if it falls from the sky we call it rain and if we play in it we call it snow. When substances take different forms, we give them different names. The terminology is just shorthand, to convey a little extra information.

There is a limit to how much glycogen a muscle can store. The larger the muscle, the more glycogen it can hold, so a conditioned athlete can store more glycogen than an average person. You cannot put two quarts of water in a one quart jug. Muscle is not a bottomless pit. Every muscle has its own storage capacity.

A person may hold between 1500 and 2500 calories worth of glycogen in their muscles, which translates to 7 8 grams of carbohydrates per lean pound of body weight. That is not terribly much, especially as muscle is rarely empty. Unless you've gone to deliberate measures, like doing a 24 hour fast or doing several hours of cardio, your muscles will be storing some glycogen.

In bodybuilding, to increase the accuracy of our efforts, we would carb deplete for several days before doing the 'carb load.'

George eats 3000 calories a day with 85% of his calories coming from carbohydrates (not an unusual occurrence). That would be 637 grams of carbohydrates per day.

George lives in Los Angeles, drives to work and sits at a desk all day. George is overweight and is getting heavier every year. George is eating more carbohydrates than his muscles can store. Thankfully (not) his fat cells have no such limitations and will happily store excess for George.

Thomas eats 3000 calories a day, 60% of his calories come from carbohydrates, that would be 450 grams of carbohydrates per day. Thomas lives in New York, walks to work, lifts weights and is in a rowing club. Thomas is not overweight.

In today's society exercise is becoming an essential, even though many people regard it as a luxury. We drive more, our work is less manual, and our time is limited. Muscles are not depleted, and eating patterns are carb heavy.

Insulin promotes fat storage, and how we eat and how much we move determines what role insulin plays in our lives. Food will dictate the insulin response and exercise will determine where the nutrients end up. You are familiar with this so think of it in lifestyle terms.

When you exercise a muscle, you deplete the glycogen stored in that muscle. If we exercise consistently, we create space where new glycogen can be stored.'Exercise' does not have to mean gym membership or even a pair of running shoes. A generally active lifestyle requires a lot of muscle activation and so depletes muscle glycogen stores. You don't see many fat guys doing construction. People who walk every day are working plenty of muscles.

Glycogen is also stored in the liver (about 100 grams), and this glycogen (not muscle glycogen) is used to fuel most of our bodies energy requirements. Liver glycogen is replenished first. Muscle glycogen pretty much stays put until that muscle uses it. Muscle glycogen cannot help if your blood glucose level drops only the liver can help with that.

In simple daily terms, it is easy and important to recall that carbohydrates stored in muscles and liver, as glycogen, are in limited spaces. Fat is not similarly limited. Sugar with nowhere to go will be converted into fatty acids and stored in our fat cells. Fat cells increase in volume to oblige our uninformed choices. Your body increases in volume, aka you get fat.

In the past weight loss diets concentrated on calories, because that's all we knew. Some people still obsess about calories. When we figured out insulin, the focus was placed on trying to limit that insulin response. Counting carbs replaced counting calories, and a new wave of diets exploded. Controlling insulin was branded in a thousand different ways to make money, which it did.

Entrenched in our calorie phobia and still terrified of fat, now we had "net" carbs to count. The advancements brought clarity, but they also yielded conflicting messages from warring divisions in the weight loss industry.

Any decent dietician or nutrition coach could tell you what I just told you. Google searches and good bloggers will tell you much the same thing.

However, there is that other tale about insulin, the crucial one that emerged as long ago as the 1950s, and yet we don't hear it often. It unravels what would otherwise be dieting mysteries: lipolysis.

We have covered this but let's look at it again.

Remember: The most sensitive endpoint that insulin has is its ability to shut down lipolysis. But what exactly does that mean again?

If you understand lipolysis, you will change the way you eat forever. You will be one of the few percent that keeps the weight off. So, let's revisit lipolysis with a mind to squaring it with our daily lives.

LIPOLYSIS (FAT BREAKDOWN FOR WEIGHT LOSS)

Lipogenesis is the creation of fat, and Lipolysis is the breakdown of fat.

> After a meal, the amino acids (protein) and blood sugar (carbohydrates) go to your small intestine where blood vessels absorb them and take them directly to the liver. The liver takes up most of the nutrients you just ate and can store about 100 grams of glycogen. Excess carbohydrates are converted into fatty acids and, of course, stored as fat.
>
> It is liver glycogen that can leave its host, travel in the blood and provide fuel for other bodily functions. Muscle glycogen cannot.
>
> If your blood sugar drops because of missing meals or creating your own food coma, being buff won't help you.

Lipolysis is not weight loss, but it is essential if you are to lose weight.

The body fat you so want to get rid of is made up of 'triglycerides'

Triglycerides are the storage form of fat and they are made up of three ('tri') fatty acids and one glycerol unit.

To lose weight the fat cell must break apart so that the four units enter the blood individually. A fat cell cannot enter the blood in

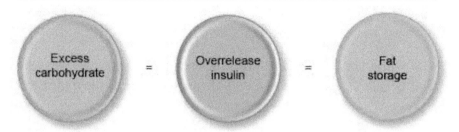

its storage form; it must be broken down into individual units which can then travel in the blood to be used as fuel. Once used for fuel, you lose weight.

However, there's a kicker: if these fatty acids are not used as fuel, they'll travel back to the liver where they'll be repackaged into triglycerides and sent back into storage. We call this, quite appropriately, a 'futile' cycle.

We need the right environment for a paint to dry, we need certain conditions for a flame to burn. In the same way, our internal environment has to be the for lipolysis to occur.

Most people never break down body fat because they are never able to do lipolysis. It would be like expecting a painting to dry in the shower.

Lipolysis is a chain of reactions. It starts with epinephrine (for you English folk, that's adrenaline) which is why exercise is a good thing; exercise stimulates an adrenaline response. Stress will also trigger an adrenaline response, and in cases of extreme stress, you'll have seen the weight drop off people in a short amount of time. Sadly, mild and moderate stress usually leads to comfort eating and weight gain. It's the big players – fear, grief, divorce, tragedy – that cause our weight to plummet.

Adrenaline is one hormone that induces lipolysis; others are growth hormone, glucagon, norepinephrine, ghrelin, testosterone, and cortisol.

Imagine a row of dominos: you push the first domino and the others fall one by one. Lipolysis is that type of reaction, a chain of events, each one dependent on the one before it. Stimulating adrenaline is not enough to break down fat, and this is where the problem lies for most people.

Mid chain we have HSL (hormone sensitive lipase), an enzyme that is sensitive to hormones. If all goes well, HSL allows for the

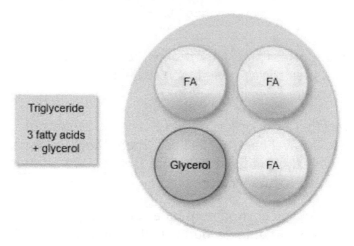

Triglyceride

3 fatty acids + glycerol

fat cell to be broken down into its individual parts. Following the activation of HSL the three fatty acids and one glycerol unit separate and enter the blood. Once in the blood, they can be used as fuel, and if they are used for fuel, we lose weight – victory!

If HSL isn't activated the chain is broken, and fat breakdown does not occur. HSL is sensitive to hormones; insulin is a hormone.

Remember again: The most sensitive endpoint that insulin has is its ability to shut down lipolysis.

When we eat a high carbohydrate meal, our blood sugar rises, and this triggers the over release of insulin. Insulin is our storage hormone, it transports nutrients into cells, when this happens our body is in 'storage' mode. It would make no sense for it also to be in 'breakdown' mode. We can only be in one environment at a time. You can't be tired and energetic at the same time, you can't be happy and sad at the same time and you can't be storing fat and breaking fat down at the same time either.

Two facts to remember forever:

- Insulin creates a "storage" environment

- Lipolysis is a "breakdown" environment

Excess carbohydrates trigger the hormone insulin. The enzyme HSL (remember: Hormone Sensitive Lipase), gets so sensitive about all this insulin invading the place that it refuses to do its job. Lipolysis stops.

It may be frustrating, but it makes good sense. When there is too much sugar in the blood insulin locks fat in storage so that the excess fuel can be used and/or stored. Why would the body allow both fuel sources to be available when there is one available in excess?

I have this heated conversation a lot in Los Angeles. Imagine a client is eating their gluten free, organic, sprouted, cereal that was massaged by a monk on a hill in Peru before being sold for $20 per pound in Whole Foods... And they're outraged that they are not losing weight. But why should they? They're gorging on carbs after all, even if they are magnificently marketed pricey carbs.

Making 'healthy' choices does not automatically mean you will lose fat.

The body from the neck down can use sugar for fuel, or it can use fat. The upshot is simple: if there is enough sugar in the blood, it will not burn fat.

If we, through our food choices, create the right environment then lipolysis can occur. If we then create a deficit in our food intake and increase our energy expenditure through exercise, the fuel we then need will come from fat, and we will lose weight.

Calorie restriction alone will give painfully slow results. Exercise alone won't work. Even being in lipolysis isn't enough if the fat released goes unused.

Lipogenesis (fat creation) is like a six lane freeway; no matter what you do you're unlikely to run off the road. By contrast, lipolysis (fat breakdown) is like a tightrope, one wrong step and you're off.

A gentleman did his first marathon, gained 10lb and came to see me. He was furious. He went from inactive to running four days a week.

Understandably his appetite increased and was encouraged to eat a lot of carbohydrates to fuel his runs, hence the unwanted pounds

As a personal trainer, I signed up for a weekend course to be a running coach. Most of the attendees worked with novice runners, organizing running clubs and charitable events. I learned a lot and was excited for day two when they were to cover nutrition. I'll never forget that the module, which should have been an hour and was completed in 15 minutes, was summed up by the instructor (an ectomorph) telling the coaches,

"Get your clients to eat well and running will take care of the rest."

I would suggest that the majority of people join a running club hoping it helps them get in shape. I would also guess that most recreational runners are not ectomorphs. When the well meaning, passionate coaches are not given the guidance that they need, then we end up with angry men knocking on the door of people like me.

Lipolysis will be halted until insulin is no longer elevated in the blood. This may take few hours; in a diseased state insulin may remain high making lipolysis impossible.

By the 1960s we knew four things for certain:

1. Carbohydrates trigger insulin.

2. Insulin is responsible for fat storage.

3. Carbohydrates from our food are necessary for fat storage.

4. People with type II diabetes and obese people have abnormally elevated insulin and an extreme response to carbohydrates.

Let's nip it in the bud and cut out all carbohydrates. Problem solved?

If we backtrack a little, we remember that the brain, and nervous system have a fondness for using blood glucose for fuel. Eliminate all carbohydrates and you may be in for a rough ride. For those who are used to a high carb diet, it's not going to feel too great at first. Most will experience hunger and cravings with moodiness thrown in.

What will get you through those first few weeks? Willpower.

We're highly motivated at the beginning of any task that directly benefits us, but studies have shown that motivation will carry you for about 2 3 weeks. After that time willpower, like a muscle, tires. It is depleted.

How long willpower works for you depends on your desire. Losing weight for a vacation and losing weight after a heart attack have very different levels of desire.

It may sound like I'm preaching that carbohydrates are naturally desirable and even essential. I personally rarely eat them and prefer to eat a lot of fat. I joke that I don't have a sweet tooth, I have a fat tooth.

The reality is that carbohydrates are not essential. In their absence, the body can make glucose itself; we call this gluconeogenesis (new glucose). The body can create new glucose by breaking down liver glycogen and from converting amino acids (protein and muscle) into glucose. When blood sugar is low the hormone glucagon (which comes from Greek meaning sweetness 'draw forth sweetness') is released from the pancreas. Glucagon stimulates gluconeogenesis (new glucose). It's like a miracle, and we should be awed by it. If you think about it for a moment, in the absence of glucose the body can turn amino acids into glucose, like turning water into wine. Miraculous indeed.

The golden rule stands: Don't ever think you can outsmart or trick the body you live in. The body is way smarter than our dumb actions.

What sets people up to fail is not the lack of carbohydrates; it is when they remove of both sources of fuel. It's the diets that require both low carbohydrates and low fat. Protein and veggies for every meal. A simple and very effective approach that yields quick weight loss and guarantees you regain all the weight.

The fear of fat, calories and now carbs lead to such diets, and I did quite a few of them back in the 1980s. It never got easier, each one was torturous, and my life revolved around my food. I always gained the weight back.

Insulin is deemed the devil, but in a healthy person insulin is only taking over when our behavior gets out of hand. Too much sugar in the blood is a bad thing. Insulin steps in to remove the sugar and we get hungry, moody and fat. But it's so important to remove that excess sugar, that insulin stops the body from using anything else for fuel. Fat breakdown stops but insulin was helping us out.

A high carb lifestyle will make weight loss impossible, and then there's the water retention. Elevated insulin makes the kidneys reabsorb sodium and sodium retains water in our body. The result for most type two diabetics is hypertension (high blood pressure) which forces the heart to work harder.

A high pressure hose is thicker and more rigid than a garden hose. In the same way, an artery under prolonged high pressure must harden to take the strain. Atherosclerosis (hardening of the arteries) can cause a stroke, kidney disease or heart failure.

For the nondiabetic, that carb feast will cause water retention and bloat. Not life and death, but it will ruin your day.

OTHER PLAYERS

Insulin is a regulator that doesn't care about a six pack and insulin does not work alone.

LPL

Lipoprotein lipase (LPL) is an enzyme (bear in mind enzymes make other things happen) situated in a cell. When active, lipoprotein lipase will pull fat from the blood and store it in the cell. LPL is regulated by insulin. Insulin makes LPL more active.

As we get older our sex hormones start to decline and we may see our body shape change. Estrogen, progesterone, and testosterone inhibit the enzyme LPL. When these hormones start to drop LPL activity increases, allowing for greater fat storage. Consequently, and very annoyingly, even if your eating has not changed you may gain weight.

Estrogen and testosterone inhibit LPL around our midsection so when they start to decline our waistline starts to increase aka 'middle age spread'. To add insult to injury, now that more fat is entering the cell there is less circulating for energy, so we become tired and hungry, eating more energy dense foods and exercising less.

LPL activity can hit your younger years too, especially if you do some hardcore restrictive dieting. Your metabolic rate is how much energy you need to exist. Expressed in calories, your metabolic rate is how much energy you need to perform all functions, from digestion and respiration to maintaining muscles and bones. We want our metabolic rate to be high. We want our bodies to be like a gas guzzling monster truck, not a super efficient energy saving Prius.

With extended calorie restriction our metabolic rate will decline. There is no reason for our bodies to keep burning a lot of energy if it is consistently getting too little energy put in. It would make no sense for the body to keep ripping through 2000 calories a day if it only receives 1000. Prolonged restriction will reduce your metabolic rate.

I have the Metacheck machine, so I can accurately check a person's metabolic rate. When someone is following a super restricted meal plan, it is common (dare I say, expected) for their metabolism to downshift between weeks four and six. About that time results slow and they either push even harder or their willpower burns out, and they quit before achieving their goal. The chronic dieters metabolic rate seems to slow down even sooner.

If/when that person quits they're left with a slower metabolism, their body needs fewer calories a day to perform the same functions. LPL, in response to the restriction, is now super active, frantically trying to store future energy. LPL responds quickly, but the metabolism recovers slowly.

Prolonged or repeated restriction will cause weight gain, even when the eating behavior does not seem to justify it.

The lowest metabolic rates I have ever tested have been with chronic dieters, and their repeated restriction makes metabolic recovery a lot less likely.

The cycle of losing weight and regaining weight is called 'Yo Yo Dieting' and what's interesting about this pattern is that the weight gain tends to show up in the upper body and arms. Girls trying to chisel their abs end up with thick waists and chubby triceps.

Intermittent Fasting (IF) is a popular and very successful approach to weight loss. One of its benefits is how it protects your metabolic rate. Intermittent fasting only requires you limit intake a couple of days a week or a portion of every day. It is the prolonged restriction that's problematic as we are very well equipped to deal with intermittent periods with no food. This chimes with my own observation that metabolisms downgrade between weeks four and six of severe undereating.

One more thing to know about lipoprotein lipase (LPL) is that the stress hormone cortisol increases its activity. For those of you that have lost weight due to stress, you know how quickly it piles back on. Excessive exercise and undereating will increase cortisol levels, and cortisol is renowned for adding inches to our waistlines. The Yo Yo Dieters probably change their body shape because of this hormone's ability to alter fat patterning.

LPL is a regulator that responds to hormonal changes and lifestyle choices that it doesn't agree with.

GREHLIN, CCK & LEPTIN

Ghrelin is a hormone that increases hunger and leptin is a hormone that communicates with the brain to let it know when body fat levels drop too low. When stored energy drops, leptin tells the brain and

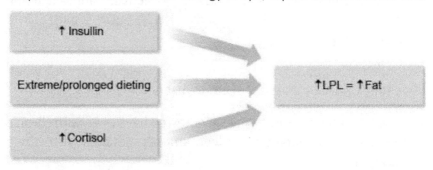

the brain sends out a signal to eat more. Appetite increases.

When body fat levels drop so does leptin. Stress can also reduce leptin levels, and this might show up as late night comfort eating.

When body fat levels are normal, so too is leptin and general eating habits. Those who have never been on a diet tend not to be controlled by their appetite. I see this a lot with men, my husband being a great example. Eats like a bird, takes half a sandwich home and pushes plates away because he's "full". The only time I see Kevin overeat is when it is food that he enjoys, and even then, he's not being dragged into gluttony by a ferocious appetite; he just really likes that food.

Not many dieters, even post diet, behave that way. Hunger is a physiological reaction while appetite is a learned behavior.

Reduced leptin levels because of rapid weight loss and/or stress can be the driving force behind obsessive eating.

Keeping the weight off post diet is tricky and understanding the role of leptin will help. If you can maintain the weight loss for long enough, then your body will reset, and your new body fat level will become the norm. If you used drastic measures to drop the weight, it's going to be a real challenge to hold on until the body finds a new set point.

A very dear friend and huge influence in my life is Mark Macdonald of Venice Nutrition, and he has always said that the key to weight loss is finding a way of eating that you can sustain forever. You may need to manipulate intake and expenditure to hit your goals but if you don't stray too far from what works for you day in and day out then you will beat the odds and keep the weight off.

CHOLECYSTOKININ (CCK)

The hormone, CCK stimulates the digestion of protein and fats, and also acts as an appetite suppressor. CCK cues the feeling of fullness and diets can disrupt CCK, which again can cause overeating.

When fat stores are normal we eat less. When we restrict our intake we disrupt ghrelin, leptin, and CCK. When the diet ends we often end up eating more than we did before dieting. We may eat more meals or eat past the point of fullness.

I have been involved in the fitness industry for over three decades, first as a competitor, second as a trainer of competitors and thirdly (and very deliberately) as an observer only. When I competed, I did 2 4 shows a year and my weight fluctuated by about 15 pounds in between appearances. The fitness industry exploded after the turn of the century, so now there are a lot more shows to compete in. It's not unusual for these ladies and gents to do eight or more competitions a year. In this era where you are only as relevant as your last IG post, there's a lot of pressure on these young bodies to compete year round.

Extreme dieting with hours upon hours of daily exercise has become the standard approach to competing. I have watched many young females fight with more and more weight gain between shows. It's the side of competing you rarely see in a post, but I've met them crying in the locker room or full of self loathing in my office.

Young, bubbly girls with bodies to die for who started competing for "fun" exit the stage with that yo yo thickness that will be hard to budge forthwith.

As sure as the sun will rise, repeated prolonged restriction with excessive exercise will cause a rebound in weight.

ADIPONECTIN

Adiponectin is a protein involved in blood sugar regulation and fatty acid breakdown. Adiponectin will react to that prolonged restrictive diet by slowing the release of stored fat. It will make your fuel consumption more efficient. In general life, efficiency seems to be a good thing, but if you're trying to lose weight, it's a big nuisance.

We used to think that fat could only be broken down for fuel in times of extreme deprivation. We now know that we can, in fact, use fat for fuel all day, every day; we simply use food to create the right internal environment and never try to mess with these regulators.

DIET DAMAGE

A rebound in weight is bad enough but chronic dieters can expect thin hair, brittle nails, constipation, IBS (irritable bowel syndrome), menstrual problems, food intolerances and allergies.

There may also be a massive shift in how your body holds water; extreme bloating is common.

A diet that involves eating the same thing repeatedly can lead to food intolerances. Women may experience hot flashes because of hormonal changes, an increase in cellulite and disrupted sleep patterns.

The consequences of dieting run parallel with how extreme and how long the diet was. Recovering from a diet may take a lot of time. I read once about the 600 day rule. Get your weight to where you want it to be and keep it there for 600 days and your body will reset. I cannot attest to the validity of this rule, but it chimes with personal experience. I stopped competing in 1996, and my body was incredibly reactive; if I ate slightly too much I gained weight, the water retention was horrid and my appetite huge. By 1998 my weight had normalized, and I didn't balloon up from one fun meal. Recovery for me was not so much about my weight as, thankfully, I wasn't too far over the mark. Recovery for me was about how I saw myself. I hated having a huge appetite, eating portions meant for a small family and being hungry all day. It's not attractive to eat like a pig at a trough, and it's not normal.

In the documentary film, 'Super Size Me' Morgan Spurlock ate McDonald's for every meal for 30 days; the resultant health issues were dramatic. It took him 3 4 months to recover from the 30 day experiment. Most diets last longer than 30 days, and they're often repeated. Recovery can potentially be a very long road, so it's understandable when frustration drags people back to what worked for them before.

The days of extreme restriction are behind us, and the trend now leans towards building a strong functional body. We no longer need to see a thigh gap or ribs to be in shape.

FOUR REASONS DIETS FAIL

This is a subject that has been endlessly available for studies and observation for decades, and we have indeed learned a lot; about human behavior and thought patterns, and why we fail at diets and many things. To contemplate why we fail is, of course, very instructive, and it's also quite amusing.

1. COMPLIANCE

Compliance; The act of complying with desire, demand, proposal or regime.

Compliance; fulfilling requirements; doing the work as clearly outlined.

Compliance is the number one reason people fail with diets. They either can't, won't or just don't do what is required. This suggests that the dieter is to blame. However, that's rarely the case.

The majority of people have the desire to lose weight. I have the desire right now to drop a few myself. Desire does not equate with action and even when it does, it does not equate with consistent action; and that is precisely what is needed in order to hit a weight loss goal.

We live with this struggle every day and not just with food. I desire a clean car (it's dirty). I desire that my taxes be done early (not happening) I really want to call a friend (months later and I still haven't).

The failure to act doesn't mean you don't care about the result. The failure to act is about the power behind the desire.

I desire a clean car vs. I'm taking a new client to lunch and offered to drive; the car is miraculously clean.

I desire to have my taxes completed vs. my husband made an appointment with our CPA in a week's time. Work is done.

I keep meaning to call a friend vs I found out my friend's mother just died, I call immediately.

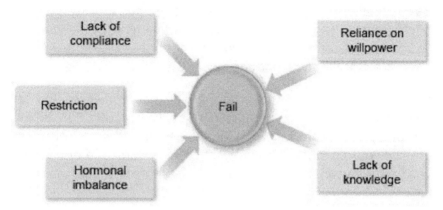

It is the power of the desire that is crucial for compliance. Think of hard and fast scenarios:

1. A dad wants to get healthy for his newborn son.

2. A bride has her dream dress and a wedding date booked.

3. An athlete has a big competition date set.

4. A patient has just been given a 'do it or die' pep talk by the doctor.

Weight loss requires more than one action. It takes months of daily action. To reduce the body fat so easily acquired there really must be a meaningful reason to subject yourself to constant daily discipline. Unfortunately, the reason we hold on to is usually weak and attached to no strict date. However, if we dig deeper and allow ourselves to get uncomfortable, we may find the strength we need.

Why we want to lose weight

1. I look awful in photographs. (Weak)

2. Which makes me not feel good about myself. (Weak)

3. Which makes me compare myself to others. (Better)

4. Which makes me avoid going out with those people. (Better)

5. I don't go out much. (Strong)

6. I'm lonely. (Bingo)

Being lonely is much more powerful than not looking good in photographs. The challenge is being honest with yourself about why you want to make a change. If you can get brutal with yourself, you are much more likely to find the power you need to succeed.

Failure to comply with that amazing diet that worked so well for your co worker might be because YOU ARE NOT YOUR CO WORKER. Do you both like horror movies, Monty Python, and tie dye? No, you are not your co worker. If you want to work someone else's plan, you better be sure you align yourself with more than just the same weight loss goal.

One diet does not work for everybody but not because you have a certain blood type or undiagnosed food intolerance that no one can appreciate (but you). Our uniqueness lies in our lifestyles, our responsibilities, obligations, age hormonal state, our body type and our personality.

A 25 year old single female with Pilates and spin memberships working 30 hours a week may get excellent results from her 30 day juice 'cleanse.'

That same lady 20 years on with two teenage sons, working 40 hours a week and dealing with pre menopause will not have the same success.

If you meet with a nutritionist and they have one weight loss plan and one plan only, I'd turn on my heel. If you choose an online program, be sure to check the testimonials and see if there are people you can relate to.

Even the worst plans can work for some people. The dinosaurs in the industry offer public weigh ins, social support, and encouragement. I would be climbing the walls but for some people this works. If you find a person or a program that connects with that real, raw, authentic reason you want to change then you've likely won before you begin.

To lose body fat you must break down stored body fat and use it as fuel (lipolysis). That's a reality nobody is going to argue with, but there are however different ways of achieving that fat burning environment.

1. Intermittent Fasting (IF) Gaining popularity and very successful.

Pros – A few uncomfortable days per week but a lot of wiggle room on the other days. Many find it easy to adhere to long term.

Cons – Difficult for those who exercise several hours a day or take medication which requires food.

2. No Carbohydrates.

Pros – Fast results. Cravings and hunger that greatly diminish within weeks.

Cons – Can feel very restrictive. Vegetarians have limited options. Socially it might be challenging.

3. Balanced meals with lots of exercise.

Pros – Lots of variety. Can work long term.

Cons – Time consuming exercise. Progress more gradual. Diligence is needed with macronutrient ratios.

These are just three ways to allow for lipolysis. One way or another you are lowering the sugar in your blood to allow fat to be used as fuel. You are controlling the sugar in your blood by either eating less food, eating fewer carbohydrates or doing a lot of exercise to use the carbs you eat as fuel. As we age, and our lives change, we may find our approach changes. When I was younger I exercised more, my nutrition was good, but I also did several hours of exercise a day. Now, at 50, I wish I had those extra hours in my day to exercise. Today my nutrition is on point and I rely less on the calorie burn.

Compliance is three pronged; it depends on a powerful desire, the correct approach and the willpower to endure.

WILLPOWER

Here is a revealing experiment. There are three groups of people, and none of them have eaten for three hours. Each group was given the same puzzle and told that the puzzle was easy to solve. That was a lie.

During the task, the first group was not given any food. The second group was given radishes to eat. Group three were given radishes and cookies but told only to eat the radishes.

No one was going to solve the puzzle, but which group worked at it the longest?

You would think that the group with no food would quit first, mainly as they were a little hungry when they started the task. It was, in fact, the group that had the temptation of the cookies that gave up fist.

Willpower takes real energy, so does fighting temptation.

The takeaway is that if you are about to enter into something that's going to call on willpower, it's best to clean your slate of any other energy sucking tasks. If you're going to set a New Year's resolution, you will have more success if you pick just one. If you decide to stop smoking and lose 20 pounds, it's going to be tough as both tasks will be a drain on your willpower.

'Focus, develop tunnel vision; concentrate on one thing, and one thing only when it comes to taxing your willpower.

Working with physique competitors (myself included) the competition preparation becomes very insular. A competitor's world becomes very small, with other facets of life such as careers and relationships being sidelined. The more challenging the task, the more willpower is needed and so your days become mundane. If your nutrition and exercise are enjoyable, you'll need less willpower to comply and you'll be a lot more likely to succeed.

I hate swimming. If swimming were found to be the ultimate exercise and proven to give me the body of my dreams, I would certainly give it another go, but I doubt my willpower would hold out very long, purely because I HATE swimming. I dislike everything about swimming, from the time commitment to how it ruins my hair to the fact that, of course, I am not good at it. I've competed in triathlons, and I say that in the past tense because I hate the swim. Do not make choices that set you up to fail. If you hate fish, don't sign up for the tilapia and broccoli challenge (and coaches, if your client hates fish don't force it on them). I can't tell you how many times a client has tried to take up running because they think they should. If you hate to run, don't run! Eat foods and chose exercises that you can enjoy. If Zumba and egg whites don't do it for you, then don't do them.

Willpower will start a task, but it won't sustain it unless you have a powerful drive behind your desire.

Willpower takes energy, and the more you use it, the more it will sabotage your ability to do other things. When we become focused on a task, we let other priorities slip. If you've ever studied for exams or had some other deadline imposed on you, you'll recall how you neglected friendships, didn't return calls, missed birthdays and let the housework go to hell in a handcart.

Here is another revealing experiment: children were given marshmallows and told if they didn't eat their one they would be given two later. The children that showed the most willpower and were able to resist had that same willpower and reasoning when they reached their forties.

Personality traits persist through life and it's wise to consider what you know about yourself.

I'm a morning person. As a child, I put myself to bed early, so that I could be up by dawn. It would be a challenge for me to sign up for a night class. If the class meant enough to me, then I would need to simplify my other obligations because it would take a burning desire and a whole lot of willpower to get me out of the house after 9.00 pm.

Willpower is the ability to delay gratification, to resist short term temptation to achieve long term goals. Willpower is the ability to override impulses and the more you rely on willpower, the shorter your fuse becomes. Willpower and the energy it takes will affect your short term patience and what you're able to tolerate.

How many diets fail on Friday night after a long week of work? Willpower requires fuel, and when you're exhausted, you're more likely to give in to temptation.

Social support can be priceless when willpower starts to wane. Weight Watchers, Overeaters, Gamblers or Alcoholics Anonymous all strengthen a person's desire to continue on the path. Today we have online communities, forums, and groups to keep us motivated and on track.

'It takes a village' is never more valid than when you take on a task that takes you far away from your comfort zone. If your goal requires some major life changes, then you might need more than your willpower to succeed.

Compliance is the number one reason diets fail because dieting is rarely fun. To succeed we must dig deep into our psyche, we have to get past the fluff and be honest with ourselves. Only in that vulnerable place can we find the strength we will need.

Willpower is not just for the big things in life. We use restraint daily. We dress appropriately when we would rather be in sweats. We order a small ice cream when we really want to guzzle a pint of the stuff.

The brain works hard to control our constant urges, and this takes fuel. I'm not here to advocate any one diet, but I will advise against one of the most popular approaches to weight loss. When a diet requires you to severely restrict carbohydrates and fat (both are fuel), it's going to become very difficult to restrain yourself from the temptations of life.

Initially, you'll be motivated by the scale, but people crash and burn at week three or four. Studies on willpower show that it carries us, on average, for less than a month. Starve willpower and it will not serve you well.

RESIST – PERSIST

What you resis,t will probably persist. You ban sugar from your life, and suddenly you see it everywhere. You break up with a boyfriend and 'your' song seems to be on the radio non stop. The men in the Minnesota Starvation Study became obsessed with food; dieters post daily photos of their meals. We fixate on the things we can't have, yet when there's no such resistance, the desire is fleeting.

Men and their cars. A man sees a car he wants, but it's close to or over his budget. The temptation is real. He'll see that car all over town; he'll research it and contact dealers. He will negotiate with himself, making bargains and agreements until eventually the deal is done, and he buys the car.

We all know that wealthy guy that's been driving the same car for over a decade. It's not that he doesn't like cars. He'd like a new car, and he has the means to buy it, but because he doesn't feel the resistance of choice it slips his mind, so ten years on he's in the same car.

That which we resist will persist in our thoughts, and resistance takes energy.

The mental energy it takes to have that negotiation with ourselves will weaken willpower. The more we go back and forth in our head, the more likely the purchase decision will happen.

Ladies, we're just as guilty. Every winter I struggle with my boot addiction. The more I try to ignore the season's new footwear, the more I see them online, and the less suitable last winter's boots become. I'll put off buying the boots, but in my head, I'll realize how much I do need them. Eventually, the inevitable happens; I buy the boots.

Losing weight requires a lot of resistance energy. The temptation will be constant, and the more restrictive the diet, the more mental energy it's going to take to stay on track.

THE COMPLIANCE SOLUTION

We understand now that compliance is the ability to stick to a plan. However, what if it is the plan that is the problem?

Pro action is a Napoleonic trait. Napoleon is said to have thought out every possible outcome for every battle he fought. He prepared and strategized and was rather successful, winning most of the time and ruling over Europe for more than a decade.

Fail to plan, and you plan to fail. Sometimes people merely haven't tried the strategy which would work best for them, and ultimately change their lives.

Remove Temptation

Throw away or give away all the food in your pantry that is not on your diet. Put your family's food in a place that is out of sight and hopefully out of mind.

Substitution

If you love your coffee shop in the morning take some time to look at what else, they have to offer. It took me a few years, but I weaned my husband off his Starbucks Panini and glazed donut and over to an egg white and spinach wrap. Making substitutions may be easier than changing the actual action.

Pick Your Battle

Choose one goal at a time. This is crucial, especially at the beginning. Don't start a diet the same week your kids go back to school and don't start that diet in the middle of a divorce or the first month of AA. It may seem like a good idea; it isn't.

Life events often go hand in hand with the desire to lose weight. Fitting into a wedding dress or ditching maternity clothes are both compelling reasons to start a diet, but weddings and babies require a lot of energy.

Too many goals will deplete your willpower.

Make A Good Choice Easier to Make

I train at 4.00 am. I'm a morning person, but that 3.00 am alarm is brutal. After my workout, I shower at the gym and start work.

To make that 4 am workout less of an option and more likely to happen I pack my clothes and toiletries the night before and put them in the trunk of my car.

If at 3 am I decide not to work out I now have the inconvenience of having to go outside in the dark to retrieve my gym bag. I then have to take out what I need to get ready for work, by which time the house is awake and I'm regretting that rollover.

Make a good choice easier than a bad choice; at 3.00 am I'm picking what's easy.

Put candy on a high shelf out of reach, keep running shoes by your bed and pre pay for the exercise classes you have to talk yourself into doing.

Make good choices easier and make bad decisions more difficult (or expensive).

If you failed in the past identify the reason(s) and strategize accordingly. You have one significant advantage over Napoleon; you know who you're up against.

The ultimate goal is to not rely on willpower. An action repeated becomes a behavior, and behavior soon becomes a habit. Habits require very little willpower.

2. KNOWLEDGE

I've been writing diets for a long time. It used to take me hours when it was just my calculator and me, doing everything by longhand.

The diet would be great and yet there was frequently a disconnect between my client's desire and action. It was a cycle. Client desperately wanting change and me spending hours creating a customized plan which they then didn't follow. I could blame the client, but the frequency spun the dial, to point blame directly at me.

All my clients had was a desire to be different, all I provided was a diet. I left them vulnerable to doubt and resistance fatigue. They were poorly equipped for the battle ahead of them.

In 2009 my clients got suited up.

Today my initial consultation starts with a 40 minute introduction on nutrition and weight loss; questions then go back and forth and then we design the meal plan. At this point, the client is engaged and understands what I'm asking them. Providing people with the information they need is setting them up for success.

Knowledge is not necessarily compliance as we all know things and do the opposite. Once we have the information we need we may choose to ignore it. We can ignore it, but we can never deny knowing it.

I KNOW that stretching 30 minutes a day is a good thing. I do not stretch 30 minutes a day, but I can't deny knowing that I should.

When people start a diet they're motivated. They're inspired and energized, and this usually lasts about three weeks. Then there's the calm of merely living the plan; this is when compliance becomes tough. When people understand the path, they are more likely to stay on track when obstacles arise. Most diets last as long as the first plateau, the first time the scale stops moving and fails to budge for several weeks. This is when the diet ends.

Imagine this.

You're dropped from the sky and when you land you don't know where you are. You have a car and want to go to the beach. You ask someone for directions, and they tell you to drive west and point which way to go. The person has more to say, but you don't want to hear it so off you go on your drive west. How long are you prepared to drive without seeing the beach?

An hour, a day, a week? Maybe that person was lying to you? Perhaps they didn't really know how to get to the beach?

At some point frustration and doubt creep in, and you stop driving. Maybe you go back to find that person to give them a piece of your mind or maybe you resign yourself and settle where you are.

Now imagine, you're dropped from the sky, when you land you don't know where you are. You have a car and want to go to the beach. You ask someone for directions, and they tell you to drive west, they have more to say, so you sit a while to hear them out. The drive is 570 miles and 100 miles are on a dirt road across a mountain range. The stranger explains that it will take you five days to reach the beach.

Now how long are you going to drive? You're going to drive for five days; you're going to buy some supplies and download a book. You will drive until you reach the beach.

Although you were eager to get started, that small investment of time prepared you for the journey. You weren't shocked when the road turned to dirt, and the mountains didn't drain your willpower; the mountains signified you were on course, closing on your goal.

"I just need you to tell me exactly what to eat."

"Give me a diet and I'll follow it."

Two statements that seem to allude to a person's determination and confidence. They're a cop out.

If you choose to follow a diet that you don't understand, you may find short term success, but you will never achieve the long term shift everyone wants.

If the nutrition coach does not (or cannot) explain their program, you can expect a quick and temporary fix at best.

Look at the dinosaurs in the weight loss industry. You get your 12 week plan, and that's. it. You buy their bars and shakes but then what? Companies that are successful because they thrive on repeat business; people coming back over and over again because "it worked last time."

My mistake pre 2009 was underestimating my clients. I didn't think they'd be interested in what I had to say, and I was wrong. Once I changed my initial approach, referrals started pouring in. Clients brought their parents, their kids, their bosses. I became more excited about my work and my clients got the results they deserved. The one thing I didn't get was repeat business, but the referrals made up for that and I like to think that's the way it should be.

BEYOND THE SECOND 'WHY'

When it comes to nutrition, we tend to have a lot of questions, but we also tend to accept short, vague answers as explanations. Here's a test to spring on an alleged expert. Act like a 5 year old and question every answer you're given. Ask until the 'expert' gets annoyed or until you're satisfied that they know what they're talking about.

The conversation may go something like this.

Expert;   You are not to eat carbohydrates?

You: Why not?

Expert: Carbohydrates will make you fat

You: Why?

Expert: Because they put too much sugar in your blood

You: How does sugar in my blood make me fat?

Can your expert go beyond the second why?

If they can go on to explain lipolysis, insulin and so forth you've found yourself a coach.

Very few coaches will take you past the second or third 'why.'

Another example:

Expert: You must not eat past 6pm

You: Why not?

Expert: Because food in the evening turns to fat

Stop right there because this dude struck out, because that statement is not even true.

Ask questions and question answers.

Don't treat your coach like the google search box. They might not have the answer to everything, but at least work with someone who can peel away the layers. There's a fine line between furnishing the client with the information they need and drowning them in detail just to appear smart.

3. RESTRICTION

If you lift weights for long enough, you will get callouses on your hands. If you walk with no shoes the same will happen to your feet. Our bodies are very capable of adapting to a changing environment. If the change is slight, no adjustment may be warranted, but when the change is great, we find out just how capable we really are.

Changes can be good, bad, intentional or made by mistake.

As a species, we've survived for 300,000 years because of our capacity to maneuver through times of restriction. Restriction can be more than the limitation of food; it may be sleep, love or a physical impairment. The prolonged absence of something we need results in involuntary reactions that attempt to take us back to a place of balance.

A severe, continuous and extensive restriction of food will cause your metabolism to downshift and run at a slower rate. You will require less energy to do the same activities. Your body becomes incredibly efficient with the limited food it's being given.

To lose weight we want to create an energy deficit, so we strive to eat less than we need. Human nature pushes us towards doing more of anything that rewards us, and some of us thrive on imposing self control that goes beyond what is comfortable. Any psychological thrill we get from starving ourselves is limited to our ego because the rest of our body is not enjoying this at all.

My observation is metabolism slows between weeks four and six on a severe calorie restricted diet. For the chronic dieter, it may hit sooner.

In the world of fitness and bodybuilding, strict pre contest diets are the norm. I've watched as progress grinds to a halt mid prep, despite 2 3 hours of cardio per day. Sadly, this usually happens with female competitors; their male counterparts have mounds of muscle that protect their metabolic rate.

The body becomes very efficient at burning fat and, despite what the treadmill tells them, they're progressively burning fewer calories for the same exercise,

Hours of training goes hand in hand with sleep deprivation/restriction. Doing hours of activity every day requires a time commitment that is not always available to us. To hit the exercise quota, we have to extend the day by getting up earlier or going to bed later so, either way, sleep is sacrificed. The incongruity between the objective and the action is that sleep deprivation is known to hinder weight loss, increase appetite and trigger cravings for sweet food.

Restriction of our social life and family time merits serious consideration. It's commendable to be goal orientated but when we do it at the expense of those around us we set ourselves up for feelings of epic failure. What is life for? Ticking boxes or savoring time with loved ones?

Life is busy and finding a balance is never easy. Friends and family become an option that we push to one side, recklessly assuming that they'll endlessly cheer for us from the sidelines. This behavior has a name: SELFISHNESS. If to succeed you need to alienate yourself from those who love you then your success will be short lived. I'd like to say that your failure will be due to you being a bad person but its less judgmental than that. If success is dependent on an unlivable schedule, then you will fail, not because of any lack of character, purely because success in the long term relies upon behavior patterns that can last longer than a 12 week weight loss challenge.

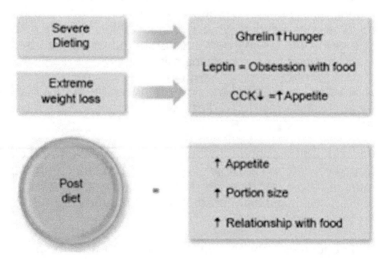

An all or nothing approach to weight loss is admirable until your life becomes selfish and unrealistic. If you're never home because you won't miss a cardio session your relationships will suffer. If you refuse to eat out because of your diet don't expect your friends to keep calling.

My condescending tone is directed at myself. My competitive years were self centered and selfish, and they didn't have to be.

Ask someone that's always in shape how they eat. I doubt they starve themselves or count calories. Their exercise is usually something they love to do, and they'll eat in a way they enjoy.

Ask someone who gets in shape a couple of times a year what they do, and they might recite a precise meal plan and cardio hours. Their plan is not livable as proved by their fluctuating weight. Strangely, the semi annual transformation gets more praise than the lifestyle commitment.

Severe restriction of any sort is usually short lived.

Long term results come from long term behavior patterns.

4. HORMONES

You can't trick, avoid, beat or override a hormone.

Like a missile, once fired it will find its target.

Like toothpaste, once out of the tube ...

You can decorate a house to look like a million dollars but if the foundation is cracked it's a tear down. You can eat well and exercise daily but if your hormonal foundation is cracked you're a tear down.

The holy grail used to be calories. Calories were the answer to everything and if we ate less of them and worked off more of them we would lose weight. That was back when calories were all we knew. Times have changed, and they have been 'changed' for half a century. Still, we have this co dependent relationship with calorie counting.

Calories are units of energy and they are relevant; they just cannot be considered in isolation. Calories are a team player, but the quarterback is:

INSULIN

Elevated insulin caused by elevated blood sugar which nutritionally is caused by too many carbohydrates. Insulin locks fat in its cell so that it cannot be released and used as fuel.

A 1200 calorie a day diet is taxing yet if the calories come from carbohydrates progress is going to be dolefully slow. If carbohydrates are properly managed, then a 2000 calorie a day diet could offer far better results.

Calories are relevant, but they are only part of the weight loss equation.

A maddening circumstance for some is when they cut their carbohydrate intake and fail to lose weight. They endure fatigue, irritability and hunger but the scale fails to move more than a few pounds. The lack of progress inclines them to quit and return to old eating habits.

Going to my tall tale of being dropped from the sky. When not equipped with an explanation these people will settle (unhappily) where they are and never get to the beach.

Failure to lose weight in the absence of carbs is common with those that are prediabetic or diabetic. If your body has been used to running off sugar and then you eliminate sugar you're initially going to feel lousy while the body figures out what to do without its usual fuel.

A high carbohydrate diet, especially when combined with a lack of exercise, means there has been a lot of insulin. Insulin resistance means that the sugar in the blood has nowhere to go and remains high even when carbohydrate intake is reduced. If blood sugar is high, insulin also remains in the blood and insulin locks fat in storage.

For a person rubbing shoulders with diabetes, elevated sugar and insulin may continue after they cut carbs. They're going to feel crappy and only drop a few pounds, which is probably water. If they resolve to continue, this situation most likely will be temporary. It may take weeks but blood sugar declines and when insulin resolves itself the body fat starts to fall off.

I started a client, who I suspected was pre diabetic, on a low carbohydrate diet. For the first few weeks, he suffered headaches, fatigue and cravings, and he lost only a few pounds. Scolding himself, he had this notion that his decades of poor eating had harmed him to the point where he would stay fat forever. This rationale led to the belief that any attempt to change was futile and he might as well go back to his old eating habits. Tough love with a dash of male pride and three weeks later his symptoms were gone, and his weight started to come down. Progress powers motivation, and now he was back in the driver's seat.

He had suffered high blood sugar and high insulin for a very long time. His insulin levels didn't drop immediately, and, despite his efforts, fat remained trapped. Insulin ensured fat could not be broken down and used as fuel. At the onset, my client couldn't use body fat for fuel, and I had taken away his carbohydrates. With both fuel sources removed, a miserable few weeks ensued.

Thankfully, my guy understood what was going on, and he stayed on course. He Lost the weight and decreased his risk factors for many health issues

Elevated blood sugar and insulin are the precursors for countless conditions, diabetes being the most obvious. Controlling insulin reduced his "risk of death by any cause" and the weight loss made exercise easier to do and more fun.

CORTISOL

Cortisol is a stress hormone, and it's a significant obstacle to weight loss. We assume that stress is unwelcome, but stress can also be excitement, anticipation, drive.

I have new clients fill out a questionnaire, which includes asking if there have been any life altering events in the last few years. Divorce, death, new baby, job change or loss, bankruptcy, litigation, surgery are all examples of stress. That one answer can tell me a great deal and show me the direction to take.

I'm not going to give a new mom who just went back to work a routine heavy in cardio hours.

Stress will add inches to your waistline and mess with digestion making you feel fat and bloated.

Exercise. and low blood sugar are forms of stress themselves. I worked with an ultra marathon runner who would routinely run 100 mile races. Although slight, her body fat was over 30%. That level of exercise increases cortisol which can burn through muscle causing body fat percentage to increase.

It would seem that cortisol is another villain, right up there with insulin. Like insulin, cortisol is looking out for us. Like parents, these hormones thanklessly do what they need to do to keep us in line.

There are two sides to cortisol as it triggers both lipolysis (fat breakdown) and lipogenesis (fat storage).

Cortisol increases HSL activity. If you remember HSL (hormone sensitive lipase) is a key player in fat breakdown (lipolysis). If you speed up the activity of this enzyme, you can speed up fat breakdown. This is a good thing for the ultra marathon runner who by their second hour has no sugar to use as fuel, but now has the bottomless pit of fat to use, thanks to elevated cortisol triggered by the excessive exercise

Cortisol increases LPL activity. If you remember LPL (lipoprotein lipase) is a fat storage enzyme highly recognized for its role in middle aged spread and other stubborn fat patterning.

Extreme stress (of any kind) can cause dramatic weight loss. In every case that weight is coming back because of LPL. Moderate stress doesn't seem to have this same effect and prefers to prompt comfort eating and weight gain.

There is the fitness competitor doing two hours cardio a day, eating low fat and no carbs. The contest is looming, and their weight loss plateaus. Panic sets in, so they eat even less and exercise even more.

The competition itself is a stress (albeit an exciting one), low blood sugar and low calories are stressors; excessive exercise is a known stress. Depending on the individual, you may also throw in relationship stress, job related stress and/or stress from poor sleeping.

Plateaus can happen for several reasons; electrolytes and phosphate levels, reverse T3, a thyroid issue where one form of thyroid (T4)

converts to rT3 aka an emergency brake. For this scenario, let's focus on the consequences of cortisol on the competitor.

To push harder seems to be the only option as the alternative would be to get out of the gym and get some rest. With a competition date fast approaching only a veteran in the sport will have the confidence to kick back. Everyone else will be flogging a dead horse (English term), and we all know how far a dead horse goes.

OK, so you're not an ultra marathon runner and you're unlikely to hit a stage anytime soon and yet cortisol may still be the one thing that is stopping you from losing weight.

If you're constantly sleep deprived, you'll have a tough time losing weight and controlling your appetite. If you've just gone through a tragedy give yourself time to recover before you start a diet. In times of stress, you can still be proactive with your food and exercise choices, it just might not be the time to restrict.

Lord knows most of us need to meditate more, stretch more, get outside more. In times of extreme stress, we don't need another spin class or juice cleanse.

SEX HORMONES

As we age our sex hormones estrogen, progesterone and testosterone start to decline. In our earlier years, these hormones inhibit the fat storing enzyme LPL. When that hormonal defense retreats we begin to gain weight and our body shape changes.

Ladies going through menopause were studied. Some ate freely. and others followed a diet and exercise. Both groups similarly gained weight!

A young girl burnt her arm and doctors used skin from her thigh as a skin graft. Thirty years later she needed liposuction to remove excess fat from the injured arm because of the hormonal influence of the thigh tissue.

'Middle aged Spread' is explained away as empty nesters being less active, no longer having to run around after a family or because of a career. Energy expenditure increases and new fat covertly accumulates.

There's often some truth in this explanation but it doesn't explain everyone. Declining sex hormones cause waistlines to expand. Women who used to have thick legs and flat tummies are horrified as their lower body weight seemingly transitions to their mid section.

In the 1970s women started to try to combat their declining hormones by taking HRT (hormone replacement therapy). It turned out that horse pee wasn't the best medication (go figure!) and many women swore off any hormone treatment because of the very real health risks that occurred.

Hormone replacement is still somewhat taboo and very much a personal choice. HRT can mean more energy, improved body composition, and a happier headspace. I knew a guy prescribed testosterone cream as middle age had caused his own levels to drop. He told me that one day he was shaving and there appeared to be a mark on the mirror, so he reached over with a towel to rub it off. He couldn't remove the mark because to his astonishment what he was looking at was the shadow of his abs poking through! Hormonal weight gain notoriously sits around our waistline and this gentleman felt that his hormone therapy had allowed him to drop a few pounds unearthing his long lost abdominals.

A women's first hint that things are changing might be more severe PMS. Although both estrogen and progesterone are dropping the sharper decline of progesterone leaves women with 'estrogen dominance'. This happened to me at the age of 47 (for many women it happens a lot earlier). I knew something was amiss when the water retention of PMS was more severe and lasting longer. I'm a happy person, but I felt a blah and my usual positive attitude was a little more forced.

Hormone therapy works for me, although it's a personal choice and a highly emotive issue beyond my scope. Two books I can recommend that helped me were 'Screaming to be Heard' by Elizabeth Lee Vliet and 'From Hormone Hell to Hormone Well' by C W Randolph and

Genie James.

It's a perfect storm. Hormones are traveling south taking energy levels with them while insulin is locking everything in place and LPL is creating new lumps and bumps that terrify us.

Welcome to the golden years of one piece swimsuits and the Hawaiian shirts that were never intended for the tuck.

That will happen if we let it.

Although the battle is real, what comes with midlife is a no nonsense attitude to life that works to our advantage. People in their forties, fifties and more are much more compliant and prepared to do the necessary work. With no expectations of an easy run, we realize we must sharpen our game and we rise to the challenge.

Social media groups are brimming over with people who have found health and fitness later in life. When pointed in the right direction these empty nesters become more, not less, active and are at last able to make their health a priority.

This strength of character grows out of decades of life smacking us around. It serves us well and can transform our mid life years more than any product, cream or therapy ever could.

CHAPTER FOUR: THE ETERNAL STRESS FACTOR

Stress is a personal matter. It motivates some, it crushes others. Some people thrive on stress while others are crushed by it. Stress can be deliberate and unintentional. There are those who are bored and lost without it and there are those who cannot function with any amount of it.

What on Earth is "Stress"?

1. calorie restriction

2. surgery

3. sleep deprivation

4. excessive exercise

5. fear

6. anxiety

7. worry

8. perceived stress

The more of these you tick, the more stress you have, and the less likely you are to achieve the body of your dreams.

The final entry on the list is noteworthy; because perceived stress is just as severe as the real thing. We spend a lot of time having conversations in our head, running over and over stories about what happened in the past or what may happen in the future. It makes no sense to do this, yet we squander much of our daily lives locked into this kind of circular thinking. It alters the reality of our 'here and now' and, combined with some others on the list, it can add very real inches to our waistline.

This sort of fretting is the bedfellow of sleep deprivation, and it is also bound up with the hormonal changes of age. Reading or listening to motivational material first thing in the morning can combat this fattening fretting. Simply being around positive, uplifting people can help enormously. Positive thinking is contagious, yet one negative person can permeate through a group with the power of six positive people. Be aware of the conversations in your head and be cautious of the conversations others drag you into.

Stress is not always a bad thing. It can come from positivity; excitement on and about your wedding day, the new baby on its way, the exam you badly want to pass, moving into that new house. It is all good stuff, but stressful nonetheless.

Over my 30 years in the fitness world, I have seen stress play havoc with people trying their hardest to get in shape. No pain no gain, more is better, the worse you feel, the better you look... The pride that comes with self punishment is quite an obstacle to overcome. It is one of the reasons I eventually chose not to work with competitors.

Take a fitness competitor or bodybuilder, especially the ladies, I'm sorry to say: They start off with a restricted diet, with little or no carbohydrates, which may work nicely in the short term. However, then they add two or three workouts a day with, at best, one day off. Now look back at our list of eight; we have 1, 3 and 4 for sure, and in most cases 6 and 7, and a frightening amount of 8.

They lose some weight, and then their body plateaus. That's when they would book an appointment with me, fabulous!

I would suggest they sacrifice one of those workouts to get more sleep and add more calories and carbohydrates, given the amount of strength training and cardiovascular activity they were doing.

Some would listen, most would not. It was not because they were stupid people. It was because they were too anxious to listen to a word I said. Often, they would come back to me after the show, with a clearer mind. Then we would make progress.

By contrast, in the run up to a competition most would choose to cut even more calories and add yet more hours of cardio. They would feel horrible and not look that great, but they would drop enough water in the last week that they might look reasonable on stage. Of course, a couple of weeks after the competition they are heavier than ever.

It is sad and not a reflection on any individual, more on the sport which applauds this type of behavior. When I first read the Minnesota semi starvation study I could not believe the similarities between the men in the study, and the competitors I worked with. The difference was that the men in the study did only one diet, while physique competitors do several diets every year. Further, their diets are much more restrictive, and they do them year after year. Cute young girls with killer bodies leave the sport heavy, out of shape and feeling vulnerable after just a few years. It's not their fault. Much of blame must be placed upon the people who guide them, who claim to be experts (many of whom are, strangely, not even in good shape).

With the best intentions, we can push ourselves too hard and move in entirely the wrong direction.

The scenario I have just described plays out mainly for new competitors. Veterans of the stage tend not to fall victim to such self sabotage.

The week before they get on stage, a new competitor is likely to be racing around like a headless chicken; finishing last minute details, slamming out extra workouts and generally panicking hysterically. The week before they get on stage, an experienced competitor is likely to put their feet up.

I would always know if a competitor was doing too much. Firstly, they are not rational; they are barely present mentally. Secondly, the obvious physical giveaway; they are unable to pee and poop before the show. A classic response to stress is for the body to reabsorb water and for the digestive system to slow down, thus creating a constipated, bloated, neurotic competitor. Meanwhile, back in the hotel room our veteran competitor is peeing like a racehorse and looking better by the hour.

I know most of you reading this are not particularly concerned about physique competitions, but I use these examples anyway, because they so perfectly illustrate the dramatic effects of stress on the body.

It's not as if we are meant to have an entirely stress free existence. Stress is part of life, and we are well equipped to handle it in appropriate quantities. However, when our bodies are inundated with copious amounts of frequent stress, then problems are inevitable.

CORTISOL AND EPINEPHRINE

(Epinephrine is also known as adrenaline in the more English parts of the world; epinephrine is generally preferred in the States.)

When stress hits the body, both of these hormones are released. Epinephrine reacts very quickly and hits the brain within seconds. Imagine that feeling you get when you get a sudden shock. Imagine driving peacefully, and you get rear ended: You are suddenly wide awake, heart racing, very focused. If you suffered an injury, you don't feel it – yet.

When these hormones work as nature intended you experience:

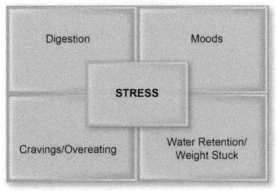

HOW DO I KNOW?

Digestion	Moods
STRESS	
Cravings/Overeating	Water Retention/Weight Stuck

1. Burst of energy

2. Lower sensitivity to pain

3. Heightened memory

4. Increased immunity

5. Regulation of blood pressure

6. Inflammatory response

It is interesting that when these two stress hormones are heightened, we form the clearest memories.

It makes sense that we would remember events that caused us extreme stress. It may be good stress, leading to a happy, inspiring memory, or it may be a dangerous situation being firmly logged in the mind under 'things to watch out for'. Consequently, we have the full gamut; from the mesmeric memory of your child being born to the searing memory of burning your hand as a child.

I have few memories of being a child, perhaps because I had a great childhood. However, I can recall when my father put me in the open trunk of the car. I was in a pushchair, so I must have been only a few years old. My dad was only teasing me, and the whole event lasted mere seconds, yet I can still see the scene very clearly. The fear I felt created a memory which seems to be lasting a lifetime.

Memories certainly have their purpose, and epinephrine and cortisol help us create important ones.

Epinephrine and cortisol work perfectly together. Epinephrine hits quickly and drops suddenly, whereas cortisol is like a rolling hill; kicking in slower, increasing and decreasing gradually.

THE PERFECT SCENARIO

Now consider this...

The epinephrine spikes may represent your four hours of sleep, waking up to 50 urgent emails, followed by that traffic fiasco on your way work, making you late. Stressor after stressor looks like those spikes of epinephrine on the chart.

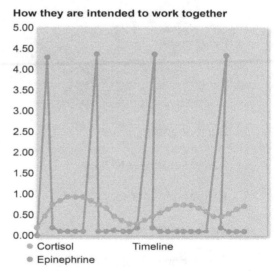

How they are intended to work together

● Cortisol   Timeline
● Epinephrine

Cortisol increases but, because the stress is continuous, it gets no opportunity to decrease. Prolonged stress equals elevated cortisol: and that means big trouble.

1. Increased abdominal fat

2. Impaired brain function/poor decision making

3. Decreased muscle tissue

4. Lowering of immunity

5. Irregular blood sugar

6. Suppressed thyroid

7. Overeating/comfort eating

8. Depression, panic attacks, anxiety, phobias, etc.

9. Possible Diabetes, heart disease, obesity, autoimmune diseases

This prolonged elevated cortisol will take you to the dark side; your mood will change, your perception will be negative, critical or suspicious. You will take things personally, you may feel angry or overwhelmed, and these personality shifts make it much harder for you to get a grip and climb out of the hole.

Your thoughts are affected, your health is compromised, and your body will change shape.

WHEN HORMONES RUN WILD

The impact stress has, is very much dependent upon your lifestyle, general outlook, and nutrition.

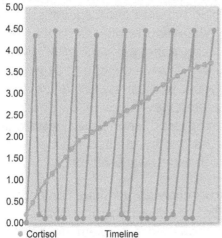

Prolonged stress
Cortisol has no time to come back down and continues to rise
Elevated Cortisol greatly affects Health

Cortisol   Timeline
Epinephrine

If you are well rested, well hydrated, eating natural, unprocessed foods (so as not to overload the liver and kidneys) and have an overall positive attitude then you are better equipped to handle stress than the person who sleeps too little, drinks only coffee and cocktails, eats out of a vending machine and sees the glass as half empty.

Whatever the nature of the stress, we can up our game and improve any situation by taking some control. By making nutrition, water, sleep and mindful thinking our priorities, we can counter the effects of stress.

How does this game play out?

When stress hits, we feel that adrenaline rush first. Adrenaline/ epinephrine hits the brain quickly, triggers the sympathetic nervous system (SNS), and we slam our foot on the internal gas pedal. Our heartbeat increases, and our blood vessels constrict. This constriction reduces blood supply. Our skin becomes pale, our hairs stand on end and we start to sweat.

On the inside, the kidneys' blood supply has also been reduced (angiotensin), and this blood also goes to the adrenals which, now compromised, start churning out aldosterone, a very fast acting hormone. Aldosterone bloats us with water and makes us look terrible, not that it cares.

In an attempt to compensate for the reduction in blood supply, aldosterone is trying to increase blood volume, and it does this simply by retaining water in the body. When aldosterone is present there can be no sodium in the urine, nada, none, not a molecule. Water and sodium go hand in hand; when water leaves the body so does sodium. When we drink a lot of water we flush excess sodium from the body and lose pounds. The easiest way to drop a few pounds is to drink more water. When stress triggers the hormone aldosterone, water and sodium are both reabsorbed by the body giving it that classic bloated look associated with excess water retention.

I've seen this too many times to count with physique competitors getting ready to go on stage. They are stressing their bodies with lack of sleep, lack of food, Lord knows what supplements and the anxiety/excitement of stepping on stage. To get the look they want, they need to get rid of the excess water being held under the skin. If they can do this, they will look leaner with more defined muscles. The show is imminent, and they may decide to take a diuretic, in another attempt to achieve that dry look.

However, you cannot trick, dodge or out run a hormone, and aldosterone is no exception. The competitor has created a great many stressors, and the adrenals are dumping out loads of aldosterone, keeping sodium and water in the body. A million times I have heard the panicked cry, "I just can't pee!" They go on stage waterlogged. Two days later, when the show is over, and they have had some rest, they look unbelievable.

This unfortunate situation is compounded by aldosterone causing the body to excrete a huge amount of potassium in our urine. When I say a huge amount, I mean a HUGE amount; we can excrete 50 times more potassium than what was filtered by the kidneys. This is never intended happen. Whereas sodium holds water underneath the skin (extracellular), potassium holds water within the muscle (intracellular). Our competitor loses the water being held by potassium in the muscles and retains the sodium which holds water under the skin. They had envisioned full muscles and tight skin but achieved the opposite.

Achieving the wrong result after months of misplaced effort is not merely a matter of superficial appearance; these competitors are also threatening their lives. Potassium doesn't only hold water in the pretty muscles but also regulates the heart. When we excrete a significant amount of potassium, we compromise the heart as well as the muscles. If somebody is badly dehydrated, you might see his or her muscles cramp, due to the loss of potassium. However, I have been in a world where the consequence was far greater; people have died due to heart failure shortly before getting on stage. It is a sad irony that their best intentions backfire so finally on their big day.

All this is to illustrate the effects of water balance at the extreme end of the spectrum but let us look at something closer to home: the vacation diet.

When we take a break from our stressful lives, we might walk the streets of Paris, or we might head to a beach to soak up the sun. While on vacation we are eating and drinking all the things we would usually avoid, like cocktails in our sun loungers or pastries in Paris but, bizarrely, we feel uber comfortable in our swimsuit, and we do not gain weight; we might even lose some. The vacation diet is the ultimate stress relieving, aldosterone crushing solution. Simply relaxing and getting enough rest can rid the body of any water retention and resolve the digestive issues brought on by a stressful lifestyle. It is worth remembering that aldosterone disappears just as quickly as it hits. In other words, you can counteract this hormone just by resting up for a while.

Going back to the brutal nature of stress, and how the body and the brain try to protect themselves: Normally, the hormone insulin transports nutrients out of the blood for storage. However, in times of stress, we do not want these nutrients leaving the blood; we want fuel available to work the muscles and the brain. The flight or fight stress response in primitive man would have meant running from something or running towards something. At such times the muscles needed as much fuel as possible to run as fast as possible. For this reason, in times of stress the insulin response is inhibited, to allow nutrients to stay in the blood.

I know what you're thinking: is this not a good thing? If insulin is not an issue won't we burn more body fat through lipolysis and therefore lose weight? That would be the case, were it not for cortisol.

In times of stress cortisol, the slower acting of the two stress hormones starts to rise and if the stress is prolonged, then your cortisol level does not have the opportunity to come back down. We are back to the trouble of 'Elevated Cortisol' meaning we get moody and fat. The trouble is, the difference between primitive man's very high level of stress, which was short and sweet; and modern lifestyles where there are fairly high levels of stress, but it can last hours, days, weeks...

CORTISOL

Insulin will block any attempt to break down stored body fat by halting lipolysis. During stressful periods the insulin response is blunted, and lipolysis/fat breakdown can be enhanced. This is because the first step in the process of lipolysis requires epinephrine, and stress promptly produces an abundance of epinephrine.

Consequently, fat breakdown may increase. But it's a never ending effort to create balance, because the same stress can also increase fat storage. There may be a little time delay between the two, but the weight lost by the stressors of modern life will always demand payback, with interest.

Cortisol increases HSL (hormone sensitive lipase), the enzyme needed to break down body fat. If there is no insulin, cortisol can increase HSL activity and thus speed up fat breakdown. This is why we see some people drop a lot of weight very quickly due to stress.

On the flip side, cortisol will increase the enzyme LPL (lipoprotein lipase). Remember: lipoprotein lipase/LPL is that enzyme that drags fat from the bloodstream into our cells. When LPL is more active, we can store more fat. Hormones like estrogen and testosterone make LPL less active, but when these hormones drop, as they do with age, LPL ramps up causing age related weight gain and middle aged spread.

Prolonged stress is like slamming your foot on the gas pedal; that pedal being the sympathetic nervous system (SNS). When this is pressed hard you feel goosebumps, your eyes become dilated to take in extra light, your hands start to sweat and your heart pounds with increased blood. Your lungs expand to take in more air and lipolysis increases to make more fuel available.

The SNS and the opposing Parasympathetic Nervous System (PNS) cannot both be on at the same time. The digestive system is governed by the PNS, so in times of prolonged stress our digestive system basically shuts down, leading to constipation and GI problems. The overstimulation of the SNS is a problem because it's the PNS that governs many of our functions. This acts to slow everything down and bring everything back to normal after the flight or fight response of the SNS. Your PNS is your 'Rest and Relax' response, and it will regulate heartbeat, slow digestion and bring blood back to your skin. You do not want to turn it off for long.

The response to stress starts in the brain and the messages it sends. Some responses are obvious, we feel ourselves blush, our hands sweat, our hearts race and we immediately feel the need to go to the bathroom. This is the short term stuff which feels dramatic but mostly won't matter a hoot in the long term. As shown above, it is healthy, normal and can be good for us.

However, as also stated, the activation of a long term stress response can be very bad for us. In fact, it can make us physically and mentally ill.

In his amusing book, **Why Zebras Don't Get Ulcers**, author Robert M Sapolsky explains how prolonged stress causes or intensifies depression, ulcers, colitis, heart disease and more. It makes instinctive sense. Zebras suffer none of these things. And zebras don't have jobs, schools, exams, financial woes or property prices to worry about.

Zebras do have passing lions to worry about, but that will be a short term stress, for all it might be their final experience of life. Zebras also don't get fat and out of shape. They look like they are perfectly content, grazing casually, lazing in the sun, gamboling in the herd and sleeping as they please.

It's the same with all mammals, except humans who have developed sophisticated ways of stressing their bodies to ugliness and their minds to places that aren't very pretty either.

ANTIDIURETIC HORMONE ADH

Stress also frees endorphins for energy, which can feel good, but it also releases the hormones cortisol, glucagon, prolactin and vasopressin.

Prolactin can make reproduction a challenge. In tandem with its effect, the stress can also inhibit estrogen, testosterone and human growth hormones.

Vasopressin is sometimes known as the Anti Diuretic Hormone. This one does as its name suggests; it retains water. In times of extreme stress that desired six pack is really not important, so ADH retains fluid in the body in order to protect the heart.

ADH is also the hormone that kicks in after drinking alcohol. When you drink alcohol, you become dehydrated. When there is less water detected in the blood ADH will be released for its anti Diuretic effect, so the next day you feel bloated.

Athletes who drop water to hit a specific weight or a particular look will release ADH. They will use all the tricks to cut water weight, but triggering that release of ADH will lead to a sudden and often dramatic increase in weight.

WOMEN HANDLE STRESS DIFFERENTLY THAN MEN – SHOCKER!

The "Flight or Fight" stress response is that sudden burst of energy, that extreme focus and increased bout of strength. It is well documented that this response is entirely different between men and women.

Traditionally, studies tended not to use women of child rearing age, and nor is it deemed ethical to use children or babies. Research was therefore limited to how men react to stress. However, it has since been found that women under pressure tend to nurture and socialize rather than run or fight. Women are more likely to spend hours on the phone talking things out with a friend, or they might join a support group for people with similar stresses. The flight or fight response is seen much more in men, and it is men who get ill and die due to stress. That 50 year old CEO who has a heart attack at his desk is, invariably, a man.

Women are capable of the fight or flight response, usually when the stress relates to protecting their children or a loved one, or a jealous rage. Mostly women release oxytocin, the bonding love hormone (Dr. Taylor), but you go after their family, and you better be ready! Increasingly, smart employers select women for jobs that are highly stressful because it is women, not men, who are most likely to come up with a calm and measured response to a stress situation, in which a man might overreact.

We all have the same stress hormones, although stress can produce different hormone profiles. Different types of stress will elicit different reactions, depending upon the individual. The extent of the response is partly due to your perception of the stress and how capable you feel dealing with it. For classic example, performing on a stage is the stuff of nightmares for some people, a dream come true for others.

What we have learned is that we have some control over how we react to stress, how we recover from stress, and how we prepare for stress.

With stress, more blood goes to the heart. Over time this can lead to a hardening and constriction of the artery walls. Think of a hose with regular water pressure and then consider a hose with high water pressure. When there is high water pressure there is more force, so the hose has to be stronger. The strength of a garden hose does not compare to the hose used by firemen. Arteries will harden to deal with increased blood pressure.

The left ventricle of the heart is the first part of the heart to be affected by high blood pressure; it becomes rigid and thicker. This is as a predictor of cardiovascular risk.

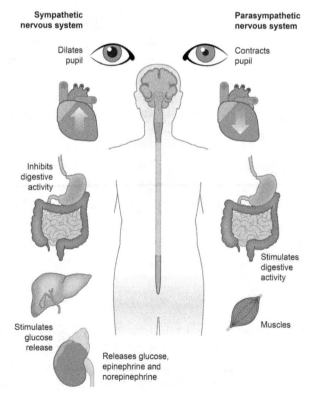

Arteries transport blood to the heart and blood vessels take the blood away from the heart to the rest of the body. These smaller blood vessels are also affected by stress; they suffer inflammation. The marker for inflammation is our C reactive protein level, which can be measured in our blood.

Where there is inflammation there can be plaque buildup. Plaque forms at the site of injury and chronic inflammation facilitates chronic plaque. It can rapidly build up in a poorly maintained body. Imagine patching a tire, and you just keep repairing it till you end up with a misshapen bulging patch. This is basically what can happen with plaque buildup. If this plaque then breaks off, falling into your system, it can create a blockage, leading to heart attacks and strokes.

Poor nutrition, lack of exercise and too much stress combine to create this dangerous environment in the body. Yet, you can be cheerfully oblivious to it. You don't necessarily feel at all worse for it. High blood pressure is known as 'The Silent Killer' for the good reason that it can go entirely unnoticed.

What you might notice is water retention; puffy eyes, a ring tight on your finger or you see deep sock lines when you undress at night. Under stress your body tries to conserve water, and you stop being able to pee because vasopressin/ADH has been released. The kidneys reabsorb water, so it doesn't leave your body. This causes your body to swell and bloat, and your urine becomes a more concentrated orangey color.

Once water gets past your kidneys and into your bladder, there is only one way it can go. This is when we see children wet their pants in fear. As adults it takes more than a little fright, but in extreme circumstances adults will soil themselves under stress. The fluid in your bladder cannot be reabsorbed; it has gone past that point. Poop and pee are excess weight and in times of stress your body may instantly dump them to make for quick physical reactions. Originally, stress involved running or chasing so extreme stress still prompts a "lessening of the load" response. It can be seen with the five year old made to stand up in class or the condemned man who is gifted with sanitary pants on the day of execution.

Stress triggers the Sympathetic Nervous System (SNS), our accelerator, our gas pedal. To gain control of ourselves we need to press on our brake, our Parasympathetic Nervous System (PNS).

One of the simplest ways to stimulate the PNS is through our breath. Inhaling deeply through the nose can stimulate the calming side of our nervous system.

That old saying "count to ten" is intended to stop you from doing something you might regret, and it works a treat. Not only does taking ten deep breaths give you time to rethink your response, but it also has a significant physiological effect. Ten deep breaths, inhaling through your nose and exhaling slowly through your mouth, will stimulate the calming parasympathetic nervous system. And this will thwart that enthusiastic spontaneous response that might have gotten you into trouble. We feel our heart rate settle and erratic thoughts clear as we enter a more mindful, reasonable state. Taking those long deep breaths facilitates a more carefully measured and appropriate response – it has saved face for me a million times.

You might be about to step on stage, sit an important exam, say your wedding vows or you may have been personally assaulted or insulted. You are riddled with tension and may sense a desire to simply not be here. Yet, in most instances, neither fight nor flight will help anything. Deep breathing will help. It brings you back from the flight or fight response of stress.

Even when aggression is in the air, when we are provoked or challenged, still a spontaneous response will rarely be our best response. It is often a shortcut to entirely losing control of a situation. Applying the brake gives us time to plot and plan, and gain control.

Heart disease is known as a big killer of men. However, even for women there is a risk, which increases with age. This is partly due to the decline of estrogen levels in women, which occurs naturally with age. Estrogen protects the heart through antioxidants that remove damaging free radicals. It is noteworthy that a drop in estrogen level can also cause feelings of panic, worry and anxiety. So estrogen declines as a woman ages and that might cause stress which in turn can also reduce estrogen; a vicious little circle. Even in a young lady prolonged stress can compromise heart health because of its effect on estrogen levels. Of course, stress in older ladies, who have less of a supply of estrogen, incurs more risk.

STRESS & METABOLISM

Insulin is our storage hormone. Insulin carries nutrients from our blood into our cells where they can be used immediately (in muscle cells) or stored as future energy (in fat cells)

During times of stress the body does not want to store nutrients. It wants physical energy to be readily available. This is because the body is still programmed to those long gone days when stress was likely to require bouts of running and chasing, away from a spear or saber toothed tiger, or perhaps towards a big tasty piece of prey or a nasty enemy who is getting away.

The stressed body has no patience with storing nutrients; storing is planning for the future, and the future may never come to pass if that saber tooth tiger gets its mitts on this body. The stressed body demands all hands on deck, nutrients included, energy resources available now, these muscles have to work as best they ever can... In today's world, there is no shortage of stress, but there is a shortage of muscle exercise let alone full out dramatic muscle exercise. By and large, there is also an abundance of incoming nutrients (food) and an excess of stored fuel (body fat). Stress without the need for movement means that fuel is sitting in the blood with nowhere to go. And excess nutrients are never a good thing. The level of nutrients in the blood is finely monitored by the hormone insulin, and if stress is continually overriding this regulator, then eventually the body will be seriously damaged. Specifically, it will end up in a diseased state – with type 2 diabetes. There is just too much sugar in the blood because the body can no longer provide it with a place to go.

Stress, and the behaviors that go hand in hand with stress predispose you to type 2 diabetes. It is, therefore, no mystery why the disease has reached epidemic proportions in the civilized world.

STRESS & CHOLESTEROL

Cholesterol is a fatty substance found in all tissues of the body, especially the brain and spinal column. It occurs naturally and is also found in animal products. However, cholesterol cannot travel on its own. It is always carried in the blood on lipoproteins. Talk of cholesterol often focuses on the number of lipoproteins in the blood. HDL stands for High Density Lipoproteins, and LDL stands for Low Density Lipoproteins; so, HDL and LDL refers to cholesterol carriers.

Think of cholesterol as a passenger and lipoproteins as a vehicle. Also bear in mind a vehicle can carry more than one passenger. Lipoproteins also transport the fat made in the liver, called triglycerides.

Low Density Lipoproteins (LDL) carry cholesterol to points of injury and inflammation, so they are deemed the "Bad" lipoproteins. High Density Lipoproteins (HDL) carry cholesterol back to the liver to be broken down, so these are celebrated as the "Good" lipoproteins. When your doctor does a blood test he wants a high HDL reading and a low LDL reading.

This is a very simplified version of events, but it illustrates the role of stress. Stress increases LDL, the bad lipoprotein and reduces HDL, the good lipoprotein. To make matters worse, stress increases inflammation in the body and LDL travels to the point of inflammation where it lays down plaque. Double Whammy!

Reduce the stress, reduce the inflammation, reduce the need for plaque formation and you reduce the risk of arterial damage and heart disease. Go one step further: reduce your sugar intake, and be aware of the carbohydrates you eat. Excess sugar (aka carbohydrates, especially fructose) is converted into triglycerides by the liver, and this fat travels on LDL, the plaque forming lipoprotein.

Unfortunately, stress and sugar intake are regular bedfellows. For many people, comfort eating is the natural response to stress. It provides the body with excess sugar which is turned into fat, traveling through the blood on lipoproteins.

You may worry that you have some symptoms, which is a stressful thought. Generally, without a check up, we never know if these processes are occurring within us. And often we are too busy being stressed to spare them a thought or too busy to take the time for a check up. Stress has its own magical way of consolidating its gains and conquering fresh territory in the mind and body. It is a pathological monster.

Bottom line: stress can negatively and dangerously impact upon your cholesterol profile.

STRESS & DIABETES

Getting back to diabetes and its intimate relationship with stress: note however that stress is not to blame with causing type 1 diabetes (sometimes known as 'Insulin Dependent Diabetes'). Type 1 diabetes is an autoimmune disease, discovered early in life and caused by the body having issues with insulin production. Insulin takes nutrients to our cells so, in type 1 diabetics, the cells are in danger of starvation. Meanwhile, the blood vessels get clogged with the nutrients the cells should be receiving. This affects the organs and eyes. The solution is to inject the body with insulin to carry the nutrients from the blood to the cells, and then all is well. Type 1 diabetes is a manageable burden, but one you carry for life; there is no known cure.

Add stress to type 1 diabetes and you have even more nutrients flooding into the blood. In other words, the stress is releasing stored fuel which it wrongly assumes the body is about to need. This stress driven increase in nutrients can lead to insulin resistance from the cells. Then the type 1 diabetic will need to increase the amount of insulin they inject, just in order to function as they did in their pre stressed mode.

Type 2 diabetes is controllable, manageable and in the vast majority of cases it is reversible and should not have happened in the first place. It is a direct result of inactivity and being overweight.

If you do not move, then your muscle cells are not depleted of stored energy. They reach capacity in a short space of time and they will remain full until that body starts shifting more. Insulin transports the glucose out of the blood but cannot take it to these muscle cells that are already full, owing to inactivity – no room at the inn, simple as that.

When there is no room in muscle cells, insulin must store the glucose/energy (or nutrients) in the only other place that can house glucose/energy: fat cells. These are far more accommodating than muscle cells. Fat cells do not have the limited capacity of muscle cells. Insulin is delighted to find these welcoming fat cells, and it starts cramming them with nutrients. And thus, the body gets larger and larger and larger...

The number of fat cells we have is pretty much set by adulthood. But fat cells are so accommodating that they will individually increase in volume, just to berth those homeless nutrients. In extreme cases we now know that a fat cell can split, creating another whole new fat cell. (This was not thought possible until recently. It could be that modern, civilized society has surpassed itself here with a brand new biological phenomenon.)

However, even fat cells can get fed up with insulin continually off loading its burdensome nutrients. So, like muscle cells, the fat cells become insulin resistant: welcome to the discomforting, body bloating, dizzying and dangerous world of type 2 diabetes.

When fat cells join muscle cells in saying 'no room at the inn' insulin responds with reinforced clamoring; meaning even more insulin comes along determined to sort out this mess of displaced nutrients. But still the cells don't want to know. They point blank refuse to take in those nutrients. The blood is being flooded. Their levels of insulin and nutrients are becoming untenable. Something has to give...

What might give – and this is a case of giving up – are the cells where insulin comes from in the pancreas. They might just burn out. Hopefully we become aware of what's happening before we reach this point of pancreatic dysfunction.

Let us return to that pathological monster, stress, who likes to play a big role in these grim scenarios. During stress, the body releases stored energy and stops energy storage. After the stress it enters recovery mode and starts storage behavior – after all the body has just burned up reserves of energy, or so it seems to believe. For two thirds of people this post stress behavior includes a considerable increase in appetite.

It is a pattern: when dealing with daily stresses, people are going through times when energy is being released and not stored. It is released into the muscle cells but hardly used. Then, as sure as night follows day, the body goes into recovery mode and starts storing nutrients as if that energy was properly used up. In truth, stocks of energy are still high, perhaps sky high. But this recovering body is bloody minded: it believes more nutrients is a good plan, it wants food, even though it's had lots already today....

It is writ large in daily stress patterns that more food will feel good. In short, wave after wave of day to day stress means constant overeating.

Owing to the relationship between cortisol and visceral fat a lot of the weight gain due to stress will be in the midsection; clearly visible in that unattractive waistline. Less noted, because it is not visible, is the fact that visceral fat is also accumulating around the organs. Visceral fat is intimately linked to heart disease and other health risks.

Again, the nail in the proverbial coffin here is that perceived stress is often as bad as the real thing. If you are a worrier and continually feel anxious about things you can do nothing about or things that have not even happened and may never happen, then you are producing the hormonal response of stress. And you are quite likely to be overeating or experiencing periods of comfort eating. It really stings if you're gaining weight and compromising your health because of things that aren't even happening. Moreover, your weight might be worrying you too now...

Perceived stress is pernicious and insidious. Pay the little monster no heed.

There is a lot of shaming and blaming around type 2 diabetes, but people are never properly taught how to avoid it, even though the science is well known and rock solid. In school there is little emphasis on exercise – you sit at a desk for most of the day, getting fat frankly

– and there is little to no importance placed on nutrition, just vague, inconsistent and nagging admonishments about eating healthily.

It is no great shock that people eat food that is handy and tastes good; the food that is brilliantly marketed or strategically positioned in the grocery store, or the heavily processed stuff you can buy out of your car window. It all tickles the taste buds but does your body no favors. Perhaps more curiously and less understood, it does your mind no favors either. Bad foods affect mood badly. However, those genuinely creative and supremely sophisticated marketing people see no need to dwell on this downer...

Fat, inactive and uninformed, we are then told that we did it to ourselves! For the apparent crime of developing a stress driven habit people are chastised and shamed and pushed towards the pharmaceutical crutch.

If nobody ever shows you how to eat well and those clever marketing people are tricking you into eating badly, then type 2 diabetes will often follow. It is natural and innocent, a hidden pitfall, easy to tumble into. Most people had no idea it was so nearby. It is therefore cruel to judge people for nurturing type 2 diabetes. It happens by way of an utterly unwitting path of mistakes. This is why they often respond to the diagnosis with incredulity.

If people are given the right information in a digestible and understandable form, they will act on it. They will make better decisions. They won't necessarily eat a consistently wonderful healthy diet, but they will damn well make sure they do not end up with diabetes – nobody wants that.

Mention should be made of people who, for whatever reason, cannot be active such as the injured, bedridden or disabled – people who are less visible in society, and perhaps literally stuck indoors. They too deserve attention and should be equipped with the nutritional knowledge they need to keep them from the grip of type 2 diabetes.

We know people learn. We know lung cancer is in massive decline for a reason: people became very conscious of the fact that it is caused by smoking cigarettes, and so they mostly stopped smoking cigarettes. It's not a proposition from Wittgenstein, just pure logic.

Ditto diabetes...

If people were taught about food and exercise – and given a reasonable amount of exercise during their sedentary school days – they would lead healthier, happier, longer lives. They would have good habits and a body of knowledge to pass on to their own children. General health could be made to skyrocket in a generation. People could easily become more active, engaged, energetic and productive – and, above all, less stressed and happier.

I think I've made my point...

STRESS & DIGESTION

Some of the calories in the food we eat are used as energy for the digestion of that food. Energy (calories) is necessary to fuel the digestion process which breaks food down into small absorbable forms. This is one of the reasons it is best we eat whole foods that have not been processed. There is a greater calorie deficit when we eat a high protein egg omelet than when we drink that protein shake. We call this the thermic effect of food (TIF) and it is a function of your metabolic rate. If you eat a lot of processed foods and drink too many shakes instead of meals, then you reduce the number of calories you could have potentially used in the digestion process.

Digestion needs energy and in stressful times we do not want to use up unnecessary energy, so our digestion slows. Because digestion starts in the mouth with saliva we may also experience cottonmouth. People who do public speaking or perform on stage may experience cotton mouth before or during their event.

We might find ourselves constipated as we tense but, as noted above, the opposite may very well happen. You may find yourself caught short, desperately running to a bathroom. Stress can bring on a very strong urge to poop. I have two cats who I adore, and they are mostly indoor cats, but I let them out occasionally. We live in Malibu which is also home to coyotes. I have heard them at night but have yet to see one close to home. Even so, we have a very high fence around our yard which I doubt a coyote could jump over. Cats, being cats, love to hide and try to escape. On the few occasions when I have looked out and realized a cat is missing, my heart has started to race, and panic has taken over me. The immediate stress response is intense. I have been known to scale and jump the huge fence, something I could not do otherwise. But before I can do anything I have to hit the bathroom.

It could be worse; stress can result in diarrhea. Water is usually reabsorbed but when there is not enough time your body will expel, ready or not. People who suffer with IBS (irritable bowel syndrome) may experience either diarrhea or constipation. The doctor may not be able to identify any one thing as the cause but stress, in its various guises, could be playing a big role, causing digestive problems or worsening them.

The stomach can be specifically targeted by stress. It has many layers with mucus to protect itself from the naturally acidic environment. However, during times of stress, the stomach wall weakens, so when that comfort food arrives the stomach simply cannot deal with the onslaught, it lacks its protective fortification. This can lead to digestive distress and even to ulcers.

STRESS & CHILDREN

When a pregnant lady is stressed it can lead to low birth weight and an increased risk of diabetes as an adult. It is now known that extreme stress during childhood can affect height and growth.

A lady from the Victorian era has two sons and loses the 13 year old in a skating accident. The mother is so traumatized over the death that she ignores her 6 year old son. She did not touch or hold her son and when she did speak to him it was only to compare him to her dead child proclaiming how perfect the 13 year old had been. The father did not interact with his child which may be a product of the era or of the man himself. Due to severe emotional stress the child grows to only 4'10".

The surviving child was J.M. Barrie the acclaimed British writer and author of Peter Pan, the story of the boy who never grew up.

King Frederick of Sicily in the 1300s wanted to know what the natural language would be if children were not influenced to in any way. This lunatic King took infants and kept them alone in separate rooms. They had plenty of food and were comfortable with good blankets, but they had no human contact whatsoever. His goal was to see what language would develop. None did because all the children died. Lack of human touch and interaction is a deadly stress in itself. Without it, processes essential to development will not occur. Atrophy occurs instead, throughout mind and body.

Lack of development is seen in children raised in severe isolation and we also see it in some adults who isolate or repress themselves. Both succumb to the stress of loneliness.

STRESS & ANGER

I am English, and the English are said to be a little repressed. A British "stiff upper lip" refers to a lack of emotional expression. Behind closed doors, I am not always sure it is a fair depiction, but at times there does exist among my countrymen and women a grit determination to rise above the vulgarity of emotional displays, even when the displays are not embarrassing or difficult in any way – even when they are fun. Opting for aloof detachment is not unlike deciding to be lonely.

A rat is given a little electric shock, just a very mild but repetitive electric shock; it does not hurt, but it is annoying after a time. Another rat is experiencing exactly the same thing, but this second rat has a piece of wood to chew on. The hormonal stress response to the electric shock is a lot less in the rat that has the piece of wood. That rat has a way of relieving its stress. Given that some degree of stress is unavoidable, we all need a piece of wood.

We all need an outlet. As children, it might be biting fingernails or pulling hair out. When people deliberately cut themselves, it is usually to relieve themselves of some other sort of pain. We may scream, we may break things, we may punch things. Women tend to call their girlfriends and talk for hours and hours (Gentlemen, this is a good thing, so let it happen). Men are more likely to go to a boxing gym, drive a car dangerously fast or gamble. We are all trying to find a piece of wood to chew on. When we recognize this, we can create environments that relieve stress. Running has always been a good one for me and playing with my pets puts me at ease. Cooking, music, massage, sex, hot baths, beach walks, mountain hikes, charity work and meditation are all good pieces of wood. Everyone has to find their own and it doesn't necessarily matter what it is – just so long as you find it.

The failure to find a good way to counteract your stress can lead to desperate and destructive behaviors. And a body that seems to be at war with itself.

STRESS, SEX & REPRODUCTION

Stress impacts on a lady's menstrual cycle and the sex hormones of both men and women.

Stress immediately causes a drop in circulating testosterone. The brain shuts down LHRH (luteinizing hormone releasing hormone) which shuts down FSH (follicle stimulating hormone) which, in turn, decreases circulating testosterone.

Exercise, although hopefully enjoyable, can also be a form of stress. The endorphins we relish when we exercise can also cause the brain to shut down LHRH. Exercise can certainly give us a euphoric feeling, but excess exercise leads to male athletes with lower testosterone and female athletes with menstrual irregularities.

If LHRH is shut down it will affect a man's testosterone and the woman's follicle stimulating hormone (FSH) which is crucial to the menstrual cycle. Enough stress from any source can cause this to happen.

The very act of sex is controlled by the nervous system. When stressed we shut down our circulating blood supply so the skin might seem gray where once we had a healthy flushed complexion. In the same way, if blood is taken away from the very area needed to perform sex then a gentleman may have performance issues in the bedroom.

Most men wake up ready to perform, with plenty of blood in that area. A morning erection is the result of sleep. During sleep we are in a relaxed state and we switch from the SNS (sympathetic nervous system) to our PNS (Parasympathetic nervous system). The nervous system takes its foot off the gas pedal and moves to the calm and relaxing PNS.

Tantric sex works with the nervous system by finding a balance between the gas pedal and the brake. If we can control the sympathetic nervous system and thereby sustain a relaxed state during actual sex, then it can last longer.

In women, the hormonal chain of events needed to have a regular menstrual cycle and to get pregnant can be significantly affected by stress. If you think of it like dominoes standing in a line, you have to push the first one hard enough so that all the others will fall. Similarly, if the hormone LHRH is not pushed hard enough then the other hormones are not released properly, and the menstrual cycle is affected.

Women do not just have female hormones; every woman has androgens (a group of hormones related to masculine traits.) Fat cells contain an enzyme which breaks androgens down and converts them to estrogen. If we do not have enough fat, then we do not have enough of this enzyme, and therefore androgens are not broken down. Now we have less estrogen and too many androgens. This is the wrong balance needed for pregnancy. It is also one reason why super lean ladies often do not have regular menstrual cycles.

All of this relates to why ladies who are desperately trying to get pregnant sometimes do not. Everyone has heard the story of the couple that tries for years unsuccessfully to get pregnant. Eventually, they give up or choose adoption. And then along comes the "miracle" pregnancy. Although pregnancy is itself a miracle, this phenomenon is not. When the pressure (stress) to get pregnant is removed, the hormones return at full strength, and pregnancy becomes possible.

STRESS & GETTING SICK

In short bursts stress will boost your immune system and protect you from illness. Your immune system fights off infection and protects you from all manner of sickness, from the common cold to serious health issues.

When stress is prolonged your immune system becomes weaker. If we keep our foot on the gas pedal, eventually we will burn out the engine. In the same way, our immune system is compromised by long bouts of continuous stress.

I experienced this myself many times back in the days when I competed. A competition diet would be anything from 10 to 14 weeks. There would be hours of exercise every day with a restricted intake of food. The drive to compete and the adrenaline rush would keep me on track and get me on stage in hopefully pretty good condition. As soon as the competition was over I would get sick.

The adrenaline response that had kept me going was no longer needed. In truth, I was exhausted, and now unmotivated with a suppressed immune system. So, I picked up every bug that was floating around.

I only competed a few times a year, but today's competitors compete twice as much and more. They are dieting and pushing their bodies to the limit for every competition, with very little downtime in between. Many struggle with much more than the occasional cold. Depression, injuries and dramatic weight gain are common, especially among novices (see the start of Stress section).

This scenario is not limited to the life of an athlete. Perhaps you too can relate to this: the vacation cold. You have been working hard all year and have been looking forward to your vacation time. As soon as you arrive, you get sick.

Similarly, there is the lady that spent months planning her wedding, the big day is amazing, but she gets sick a day or so into her honeymoon. As the stress is lifted, her thrashed immune system is exposed and vulnerable.

The excitement, the drive, the anticipation, the heart pounding and anticipatory energy we feed off during these times leaves us as soon as the event is over. It leaves us with a suppressed and vulnerable immune system. Physiological stress is not always caused by the bad things in life; it can be the fun things too, from vacations to weddings, performances, achieving goals and hitting targets.

Stress may be the pressure we put on ourselves to succeed. It can be a motivator and a catalyst for excellent outcomes. However, long lasting and continuous stress is always a problem, perhaps leading to depression, anxiety, sickness and more serious health issues.

Think of the highly motivated businessman that drops down dead before his time, leaving all his wealth to his stress free wife. Despite the death of a partner being a factor in shortening life expectation, the wife does, on average, live for another 12 years.

STRESS & SLEEP

There are five stages of sleep, occurring during a cycle that lasts about 90 minutes. Stages one and two are light sleep where you might wake up at the slightest thing. Deep sleep comes with stages three and four. REM (rapid eye movement) is where the fun begins. The brain becomes very active, even more dynamic, and using more energy than when it is awake. (Overall the brain uses approximately 25% of our energy.)

Sleep shuts off our stress response, and glucocorticoids only start to rise during REM sleep. We might wake during REM – especially if it is a bad dream – but usually we do not, and usually, it is not for long. The simple point is one we all know but do not always act on: the more uninterrupted sleep we get the more we can recover from stress. Sleep is the every day constant enemy of stress.

After a few days of not getting enough sleep out functions are impaired, we make mistakes, we become irritable, we retain water, and we eat a lot more – we are stressed. We have all experienced waking up from a much needed sleep and feeling so much better. There are times when just one good night's sleep creates a whole new world.

Stress does fight back, sometimes waging nightly battles with sleep. We have all experienced stressful situations keeping us awake at night, perhaps all night. On such occasions, the SNS (sympathetic nervous system) stays in full effect, and our mind runs riot precisely when it is time to sleep. Relaxation and distraction are the obvious weapons for fighting this. However, they are not necessarily easy for the stressed mind to call up.

Remembering that right now, as you lie there in the dead of night, there is probably nothing to do or decide about whatever is stressing you. Sometimes that one thought is all we have in our arsenal, and sometimes it is enough.

Our body can go several weeks without food, it can go only a few days without water, and it will die without sleep.

In my nutrition business lack of sleep and lack of weight loss became such a frequent occurrence with my clients that I formulated a natural sleep supplement. It was this one product that led down the rabbit hole of a new business as a retailer on Amazon. Sleep Formula continues to be one of our best selling products. You can find it at www.theshrinkshopsleep.com or find all our products at www.theshrinkshopamazon.com

STRESS MANAGEMENT

When we're super stressed the last thing we want to hear is how we "have to relax." We roll our eyes and promise ourselves we will relax at some indeterminate point in the future. We keep our foot on the gas, our thoughts become irrational, and we become more irritable. The reality is we really do need to calm the hell down.

We rely on a network of feedback loops. Feedback loops are messages that travel around the body giving out information about what is going on. When our body is too low on fat, the brain will be notified. The brain reacts by slowing the breakdown of fat for fuel. And it conveys the message that the body needs more fuel; hunger alert, your appetite may increase, weight loss may slow, you may even gain a few pounds.so we may add a few pounds.

Such feedback messages do not pay the slightest attention to what you may want. You might be super lean, but you want to be even leaner. That feedback message will not pander to your desire. It is concerned with homeostasis and balance.

When we are sleep deprived and low on energy, the message may be that we need more energy. This could easily cultivate a sweet tooth because we will want energy dense foods which our brain can feed off pronto. It is well known that those who do not sleep enough eat a lot more than well rested folk.

How we handle stress depends upon how we handle these feedback messages and indeed what those feedback messages will be. It's a bit of a communication loop, and you want to be in control of the signals. This is where stress management techniques are vital.

It is the same stress hormones that respond to any stress, but it is not merely an on/off response. How hard these hormones hit depend on how well we are prepared. For those who handle stress well, the hormonal impact might be negligible, compared to the same stressor placed on a tightly wound individual.

Stress management techniques can control the SNS, our gas pedal or our flight or fight response. Again, remember the rat that had some wood to chew on was better able to deal with the mild electric shock. In a similar way, stress management is both preemptive and reactive, and is best started before the stress even arrives.

PREPARATION

Who are you? Do you lose your mind when your car won't start or when you sleep through your alarm? Does breaking a nail ruin your day? Do you live in the reality of the glass being bone dry?

Or, are you calm and collected when your roof falls in landing on the new computer you borrowed from a friend? When that lightning bolt missed you by a hair did you think it was "cool" or when that security guard made you miss the last flight did you make the most of a night in a new city?

Stress is all about perception, and perception is personal. Perception is not, however, a fixed state.

How we deal with stress has a lot to do with our personality type and even more to do with how much control we believe we have. Feelings of control and confidence puncture the power of stress. The rental car breaks down in a foreign country, but you are a mechanic and speak the language. The control and confidence you feel just made that stressful situation a lot more manageable.

We respond differently to a stress we were expecting. A final exam or a stage performance is a little different to a car accident, or a karaoke mike being thrust into your hand. Control and confidence are clearly linked to preparation, and the ability to prepare is a stress management tools we can all use. We know that Napoleon went over every possible battle scenario before going to fight and we know of athletes who visualize a race over and over as part of their training.

Feeling you are in reasonable control of the situation will reduce any stress that situation can generate in you. When you lose your biggest client and your business comes to a grinding halt, your mind might run away: how are you going to pay the bills? Are you going to be homeless? Will you be able to pay the bills and feed your family? If, however, you have been in the business for some time you will be less likely to panic. You may even have a plan for just this situation and decide to enjoy some downtime.

Losing weight is no different. It is stressful and does not always go according to plan. Understanding the plan you are following will provide you the confidence you need to continue. Knowing how to order when the food you wanted is not available will give you the control to stay on track. Organizing your meals or looking at a menu before hitting a restaurant might prepare you well enough to avoid diet related stress altogether.

Stress is a lot more manageable if you know it is the precursor to something greater. Ladies, if you have ever had a facial peel, you know those three or four days of lizard like skin are totally worth the end result. If you were not forewarned, you might go crazy with panic. Knowing what is going to happen can reduce stress to zero. OK, there are some really ugly days on the horizon, so you plan some housework, collect some DVDs and hunker down – it's quite calming, not stressing at all. In short, the very same situation will elicit completely different reactions depending entirely upon what you are expecting.

It is not good to focus on an improbable stress. I live in Los Angeles and I know one day the big one is going to hit. I was there for the 1994 Northridge earthquake, so I know what we can expect. To spend my energy dwelling upon the future day when the ground will shake does not benefit me. There is something to be said for buying some flashlights and having an emergency plan, but to remind myself daily that I live on a fault line – to dwell upon this known, established fact at all – is not going to help anything. It's certainly not going to avert or minimize the earthquake – that fault line couldn't care less what is running through my head. If I think about a future earthquake only one thing happens; some anxiety gets added to my day.

The same goes for the hypochondriacs who see sickness in every pimple and fear contagion with every handshake. There is a possibility that a pimple is going to be the death of you, but I wouldn't go betting the farm on it.

Generalized worry is another layer of stress we add to our lives. When we are not well rested or are over worked or under fed, the worry seed takes root. It is estimated that over 85% of our thoughts are not based on reality. The vast majority of the chattering in our heads is just stories we create.

If a worry is genuine to you, then take the time to prepare. If you worry about your work, increase your value or create a new path. If you worry about the diabetes in your family, then take steps to educate yourself and learn how to avoid it.

The greater the chance of something happening the more motivated you are to prepare for it. The big one may or may not hit in my lifetime, but we're being told to expect a major storm in the next few weeks. I admit I have not yet bought flashlights, but we did go out and buy sandbags to protect our home from the forecasted rain. The way you prepare for something stressful depends on how probable it is.

The boss you dislike may or may not fire you, but there is a solid chance that your kids are going to college, making it more likely that you create a college fund than a new career plan.

Elevated and prolonged stress will not give you the body, health or energy you desire.

- Identify the stressors you can control.

- Identify two or three ways you can minimize them.

- Write these action steps down and live the plan.

Keep the plan close by so that when you do get overwhelmed, you can refer back to it and feel more confident and in control.

I learned this technique from Brian Tracy, a motivational business guru whom I have listened to for decades. In his work he suggests picking the worst thing that could happen in your professional life and in your personal life. For me, at that time it was the gym I worked at closing and losing my husband.

Neither event was probable but what could I do to take better control of my future.

1. I took control of my husband's eating habits and booked regular blood work to keep tabs on his health.

2. I took on more clients outside of the gym. Not something I wanted to do as it meant driving in LA traffic, but with this new frame of mind it proved quite enjoyable.

The gym is still open, and my husband is still smiling. Yet being proactive brings with it a sense of power and a sense of peace.

WHAT TO DO, WHAT TO DO?

The stress response is there to protect us. It's not there to make us look pretty or give us a six pack. As I say, the stress response is like slamming your foot on the accelerator. With multiple stressors that last over an extended period of time, things start to go awry:

1. Loss of muscle mass and an increase in body fat, especially in the abdominal area.

2. Hormonal dysfunction including our thyroid and sex hormones.

3. Water retention and skin that starts to look dull and lifeless.

4. Digestive problems.

5. Cravings and irritability.

6. The inability to sleep, leading to more irritability and bad choices.

7. A compromised immune system, you become more prone to getting sick.

8. Depression and perhaps paranoia, which just makes the whole thing even worse.

THE ANSWERS

PREPARATION AND CONTROL

We underestimate ourselves when we get carried away in stressful situations. And we forget that every situation, every emotion, is temporary. We will not always be happy, and we will not always be sad or angry or scared or overwhelmed or panicked... Taking a minute to honestly recognize that what we are feeling at this moment is not going to last can genuinely diminish the power of stress enormously. This is especially true for the extreme emotions of anger and fear.

Brian Tracy taught me to consider not only what are the worst things that could happen in my business and personal life, but also to consider what I could do this very day to lessen the chances of these dreaded events. This is a great life lesson, but better still, it yields excellent results in the face of stress.

As I said, at the time I was listening to Brian Tracy (I love to listen to my books) the worst possible things were, in business, the gym that I had worked in for 22 years might close its doors, and the worst possible thing, in my personal life, was ever lose my husband, Kevin.

I recognized my two greatest fears, and I found two areas where I could take control. As shown previously, preparation and control bring peace of mind to any stressful situation, even if the stressful situation is not yet real or even probable.

ACTION

Identify the real, potential and possible stress factors in your life (business and personal).

Take just 15 minutes to write down what you can do today to lessen the impact or avoid altogether the stress that concerns you.

Performing this action gives us a confidence, a feeling of power. Being preemptive is the key here. If we just wait for the stress to hit, then we might be too overwhelmed to think straight. Usually I would not recommend worrying about things that haven't happened yet – as we know this is, in itself, a stress – but to formulate a plan of defense which gives confidence will allow you to set that worry to one side.

Think again of Napoleon, mapping out every possible outcome for every battle as he prepared for each. You may have heard the saying, 'failing to plan is planning to fail'. Napoleon indeed saw it that way, and he was, arguably, the most successful military man in history. He instinctively knew preparation was the way to overcome stress and fight with a clear head.

YOUR OWN THANG...

Everybody has something in their life which helps them decompress. Whatever it is for you, it eventually brings you to a calm, clear place.

For me: I may be lying on the beach, a million thoughts racing through my head, total chaos in my mind with one thought bouncing off another one, but then, after a few minutes I feel that internal drop, like my body just melted into the sand and I am calm, just relishing being here.

We all have a way to get to this place of internal calm. For some it is massage (not me, I hate massages), a long bath, a quiet walk around the neighborhood, a phone call to a friend or a prayer. It may be cooking (also not me) or listening to music, playing with a pet, a funny movie, a sunset or watching your child sleep. We all – including the biggest and baddest and busiest of as all – can find this place. And I cannot stress enough (excuse the pun) how vital it is to visit it.

Whatever it is for you, I strongly encourage you to embrace it frequently. It needn't be that two hour massage, it can be just sitting in your car for five minutes and looking at photographs of your family, listening to your favorite song or making a quick call to a friend.

Women take this instruction better than men, but as we have already noted, women handle stress better than men too.

WHAT ELSE MIGHT WE DO?

Sleep deprivation is a stress, so it is good to prioritize sleep over that to do list nagging at your evenings. The body is forgiving about sleep; it lets us play catch up. If we have a long week with not enough sleep, we can balance it somewhat by getting more sleep on the weekends. Personally, I'm not a fan of sleeping in, because it just throws my sleep patterns off for days to come. However, if you are exhausted, and your body clearly wants to sleep in – needs to sleep in – then do it. Sleeping in is not necessarily a waste of time. It might be time very well spent indeed; time invested in the health of your mind and body, and therefore likely to enrich your quality of life. I prefer to go to bed a little earlier, but I know that goes against the grain with some people.

I can hear that little voice in your head screaming at me, telling me how busy you are and how long your days are. I'm not talking about going to bed hours earlier, I'm asking you to consider maybe just going to bed 15 minutes earlier. Monday through Friday an extra 15 minutes gives you 75 minutes overall and that can impact very pleasantly. As a mother, it might mean everybody in the house ending their day 15 minutes earlier so that you can do the same, but so be it.

FOOD

Of course, we put less stress on the liver and kidneys if we eat less processed food; better still, no processed food. Our organs don't have to work so hard if they don't have to deal with all the artificial additives and fillers in packaged food. In times of stress let's not add to it by making our organs have to work harder.

WATER

Get into the habit of drinking at the very least one ounce of water for every kilo of body weight (or half an ounce for every pound of body weight). A drop of 2% in hydration equals a 20% drop in energy. Water may not have calories, and we may not think of it as a fuel, yet hydration is crucial to energy. When we don't have enough water in our blood volume we trigger ADH to keep more water in the blood, which knocks the system out of kilter (see previously). However, if we drink enough water the body doesn't have to do this, and we lessen our internal stress, look better and have more energy.

Strangely, drinking more water can be quite a challenge for some people. When you first wake up, drink four to eight ounces of water as soon as possible. Drinking first thing in the morning can make you to want to drink more throughout the day.

For those of you who love structure, start by drinking four ounces of water every two hours, do this for a week, then increase it to six ounces of water every two hours the following week, then increase it to 8 ounces... Before you know it, you'll be at 64 ounces a day, which is still not enough but it's a very good start and far more than most people drink at present.

CHAPTER FIVE: TIME TO GROW UP

Women, periods, puberty, PMS, pregnancy, postpartum, perimenopause and menopause.

Men just get old.

Not exactly true, but women deal with fluctuating and declining hormones throughout their lives. Every woman knows the effect hormones can have on her body, her energy, and her thoughts.

As teenagers, both boys and girls get a hormone hazing; acne and moods spare no one (and no parent). However, it is the girls who, seemingly overnight, get a disorientating wake up as they enter the state of womanhood. One day they are carefree, playing dress up in mom's shoes, the next day they're having an uncomfortable conversation with the lady wearing the shoes.

Girls enter those awkward pubescent years with about 6% more fat than boys the same age. Girls continue to get fat, and by the time they exit puberty, they have 50% more fat than the boys of the same age. Boys, on the other hand, start off in a better place than the girls and lose fat during puberty.

Hormones are running riot in the young bodies of pubescent children. Boys have more testosterone, which increases their lean mass and so reduces their percentage of body fat, while girls have estrogen and progesterone, adding curves and the need for a training bra.

Bad skin, the onset of a girl's menstrual cycle and mood swings make this a fun time, and hormones can be blamed for all of it.

Of the girls and boys who become obese as teenagers, 75% will be obese as adults. There is most unquestionably a genetic factor, but this statistic is also a function of exercise and food habits, and these are, in turn, a function of parental influence.

It makes me grateful for being the age I am. Early in my teenage years, I didn't pay any attention to what I was eating. Whatever was put in front of me is what I ate. The microwave was just being introduced and I don't recall any fast food, unless you count the ice cream truck.

The food I ate was unprocessed, the servings I ate were determined by my parents, and I was a very active child, involved in many sports and there was no video games or TV in my room.

The kids today have it tough in many ways. Fast food everywhere, colossal portion sizes being the norm, more computer time, less physically active time, parents busy working longer hours; it all leads to more energy dense food coupled with less energy burning activity which makes weight gain unavoidable.

As girls leave puberty, they become women, and the hormone cycle begins. They will have to deal with this for the next four decades.

At birth a woman has 100,000 to 400,000 eggs in the form of follicles. Follicles ripen, and one turns into an egg. If that egg is fertilized, pregnancy may follow. If the egg is not fertilized, the cycle starts over again.

PMS (Pre Menstrual Syndrome) is the result of the imbalance between estrogen and progesterone. If estrogen dominates, the female may feel anxious. If progesterone is too high the female may feel depressed. The balance depends on how much of each hormone the ovaries produce and how well they are broken down by the liver and excreted by the kidneys.

Stress, sugar, alcohol, and medication can challenge the liver and the kidneys, making PMS symptoms worse.

Fatigue is one of the most common complaints around this time of the month. One of the reasons fatigue sets in is because the female body becomes very insulin sensitive. Remember that insulin is your storage hormone, triggered by too many carbohydrates in the blood. The result is that insulin removes the carbohydrates from the blood and puts them into storage (i.e. fat). When carbohydrates are removed from the blood our blood glucose level drops, and so does our energy. The natural response to low blood sugar is hunger and cravings. Another major complaint with PMS is sugar cravings and overeating.

When PMS causes insulin sensitivity, women become more susceptible to the energy crash of low blood sugar after eating. I can certainly relate to the constant feeling of hunger and fatigue at this time of the month, but the biggest mistake would be to give in to the cravings and to eat something sweet. That sugary fix will make the whole situation even worse. It's better to snack on nuts, cheese or a protein source, in fact, pretty much anything but sugar. Eating carbohydrate dense foods will spike insulin. Insulin will do its thing, crash your blood sugar and lock fat in its storage cell. Cravings will follow, and the vicious cycle of eat, crash, crave will persist.

Ladies be aware that this is going to be a part of our life for the majority of our life, so create good habits asap. The week before your period try to get more rest, stop the processed food and booze (as they challenge the liver and kidneys), cut the sugar (read your labels because it is everywhere) and hit the gym for a little endorphin high.

The high estrogen will stimulate the adrenals and will reduce urination. As if we didn't feel bad enough, during our period water is being reabsorbed leaving us uncomfortable and bloated. About 40% of women experience this. I have found that dandelion root tea is helpful but not the perfect answer. Again, if you are eating sugar, processed foods and not sleeping enough, you will make the situation worse, and water retention can feel and look worse than fat.

WHEN THE PARTY'S OVER

How we age is a function of how well we handle stress.

By the age of 70, we might expect to have only 70% of the muscle we had as a 28 year old and our sense of taste and smell will have dropped dramatically.

As we age, we have less hydrochloric acid (HCL), so we do not digest or absorb our food as effectively. This can leave us deficient in certain nutrients, especially iron, protein, and B12. Iron and B12 have a role to play in energy, so when they are low, we become tired, experiencing fatigue which a sound sleep doesn't remedy.

At this stage in the game, we're unlikely to pull an 'all nighter'.

I'm not sure when it happened, the age at which I stopped staying out late several nights a week. I don't recall being tired in my 20's, even into my mid 30's I was going strong with a full social life and getting by on five hours of sleep. At some point after that, it all changed.

Aging is nature's way of stopping us from making fools of ourselves. Right about the age when we lose the urge, and the energy to party is right about the age when, if we did keep going, we would embarrass ourselves by being that awkward elder in a room full of 25 year olds.

We move from getting home when the sun is coming up, to afternoon BBQ's that end before the sun goes down. We move from a girls' night out to spa days. This natural progression of aging is subtle and yet, in this case, kind.

Late nights and cocktails truly stress our bodies. We are well equipped to handle these stressors in our twenties and thirties, but there is still a price to pay.

ALCOHOL

"The cause and the solution to all life's problems." – Homer Simpson

Two thirds of adults in the USA drink alcohol, the average consumption being 2.65 gallons of pure alcohol a year.

This sounds like a lot, but there was a time when alcohol was an essential part of life.

Western civilization, for over 10,000 years, had a water supply that was not safe to drink. Alcohol was at least clean and served throughout the day. Consider the fine art of the Renaissance or Classical Rome or Greece; there is always a goblet of wine to be seen. Europe and beyond was a very merry place for quite some time.

In the Far East, they figured out how to boil water to make it safe to drink. In Asia tea was more popular than alcohol. The Eastern world saw two gene pools develop and this is still in evidence today.

Acetaldehyde dehydrogenase is needed to breakdown alcohol. If this enzyme is not produced, or not working efficiently, then alcohol is not broken down and becomes toxic.

In the West, if you had a problem with acetaldehyde dehydrogenase you would not have survived. Over the generations, a single gene pool survived; those who could break down alcohol in their liver.

In the East they were drinking tea and boiled water, so even those who could not tolerate alcohol were able to survive and breed. Two gene pools developed, those who could breakdown alcohol and those who could not. It is not uncommon to meet someone of eastern descent who cannot tolerate alcohol at all. They will flush and become very ill as the alcohol is toxic to them. Go out with a European and this is unlikely to happen.

Modern day medicine has used this to some people's advantage, and the alcohol addiction drug Antabuse works by inhibiting the enzyme acetaldehyde dehydrogenase, causing those who are on it to get violently ill if they drink alcohol; like an instant and hellish hangover. The hope is that feeling sick will kill the urge to drink alcohol. It is a neat idea that is sometimes able to help.

Interestingly, women have less of this enzyme in their stomach, and so they metabolize alcohol at a slower rate and will get sick quicker. Guys don't expect your lady to keep up with your drinking, or you might be holding her hair off her face as she hurls in defeat.

Older men have less ADH, as noted at many a wedding or Christmas party.

Menopausal women become lightweights, and suffer worse after effects, whereas heavy drinkers likely have more ADH than is normal, giving them the annoying ability to be bright and breezy the morning after.

"Oh God, that men should put their enemy in their mouth to steal away their brain." – William Shakespeare

EXCESS

Alcohol, unlike food, cannot be broken down and stored. Alcohol is permeable in both water and fat, which means alcohol can go straight through the wall of the stomach with no digestion necessary.

Alcohol is converted into acetaldehyde, which is toxic and therefore makes you sick. Acetaldehyde is broken down by the aforementioned enzyme, acetaldehyde dehydrogenase and is converted into acetic acid radicals.

Alcohol must be completely broken down by the liver, and the liver will break alcohol down before it breaks down anything else. Alcohol will be broken down before fat and, with the stress of continuous alcohol, fat will build up in the liver, and the liver is not meant to store fat.

When there is an excess of alcohol the liver will call on the MEOS system (Microsomal Ethanol Oxidizing System) to help out. The MEOS system breaks down things like medication, Tylenol, anesthesia and, strangely, broccoli. If the MEOS system is busy with alcohol, then it is not able to deal with these other substances, and thus they can become toxic.

If your medication tells you not to drink alcohol it is not because they don't want you to get loaded; it is because you may not be able to break down the medication safely. There are far too many accidental deaths when people mix meds and booze. It is often assumed that these deaths must have been as a result of partying to excess but, in truth, it might be purely accidental as the liver tries to break down a long, steady diet of alcohol with some pills mistakenly thrown in on top.

Your liver cannot break down alcohol more quickly just because you are drinking faster. Your liver will break alcohol down at a steady rate, and when we consume too much for too long the liver gets backed up, and everything else that needs to be broken down stays intact and potentially toxic.

Given this knowledge, it's probably also a good idea to listen to your doctors when they tell you not to drink before surgery.

Excess alcohol may temporarily make you feel fabulous, but prolonged excess can lead to thin arms and legs because of muscle loss, a swollen belly caused by a swollen liver, and even a big nose and possible hair loss. Attractive, not!...

THE MORE COMMON PRICE TO PAY

Alcohol consumption can be a life or death stress on the body. Over time and prolonged alcohol abuse, healthy liver tissue is replaced with scar tissue which stops the liver from functioning properly. Blood flow is blocked which affects the breakdown of nutrients, hormones, and medications. There is no cure for cirrhosis of the liver.

We may handle alcohol differently, but all of us who do drink can expect to, at some time or another, experience the following...

1. The Hangover. Water is lost from the cells, especially the brain cells and, as these cells start to rehydrate, we get that hangover headache.

2. Water Retention. The sick joke is that, with alcohol, you get both dehydrated and then bloated. There is a hormone call ADH (antidiuretic hormone) which, as the name suggests, does the opposite to a diuretic. It makes you hold onto water. Alcohol temporarily inhibits ADH which means that you can get dehydrated. Post alcohol, the ADH hormone kicks back in with a vengeance. It rehydrates the body big time, causing us to swell in all sorts of unwanted places. Post party you can expect puffy eyes, rings that are too tight on your fingers and sock lines around your ankles.

3. Poor Eating Behavior. When we drink alcohol, there comes the point where our taste buds become dull. I doubt that you have experienced your best meal ever whilst drinking. Meals are often unmemorable simply because you failed to taste them. Your dulled taste buds may cause you to overeat as you chase the taste. Your fluctuating blood sugar may also cause you to succumb to your sweet tooth or fast food craving.

4. Weight Gain. We all know those fancy cocktails are loaded with sugar and calories, but there is a bigger reason that alcohol causes weight gain. We have talked a lot about lipolysis, the breakdown of fat for fuel. High carbohydrates will trigger the hormone insulin which will shut lipolysis down. Declining estrogen and testosterone slow down lipolysis and so does alcohol consumption. If the liver is breaking down alcohol, it cannot be breaking down fat at the same time.

To give you a rough idea of how that looks, two vodkas in three hours can reduce lipolysis by 75%. You can do your own math but if two vodkas have that much impact, what does four vodkas do, or a bottle of wine or three beers do you for you?

The point being; alcohol slows down the breakdown of fat (lipolysis) in a major way. This brings me to a widespread conversation; the debate about which is better – the person who has a couple of drinks per night versus the person who drinks more but drinks just one night a week. The argument might be that alcohol every day is slowing down lipolysis every day whereas drinking more alcohol once a week just throws lipolysis off for that day; and meanwhile lipolysis can be active throughout the rest of the week.

I was talking about this in one of my seminars, and a lady who had attended left me a scathing Yelp review, accusing me of promoting binge drinking! I will therefore leave you to come to your own conclusion. I will only say that alcohol consumption causes weight gain by the calories in the drink, the food we eat being more likely stored as fat, and our diminished ability to break down fat.

SUGGESTIONS, NOT SOLUTIONS

1. Do not drink on an empty stomach. The small intestine is more effective at absorbing alcohol so the longer we can keep it in the stomach the better. If we have a reasonably full stomach, we can keep the valve between the stomach and the small intestine locked down.

2. Drink water with every hard drink. This will help to limit dehydration and make the next day a bit more bearable.

3. Avoid carbonated drinks as they speed stomach emptying.

4. Do not take Tylenol as it is broken down by the MEOS system. Tylenol is hard on the liver, especially when combined with alcohol.

SLEEP

I did not really value sleep until I hit my forties. Thinking back, I trained every day, did a business degree while working part time, lived in three countries, competed and had a pretty active social life. I know I saw many midnights, and I have always woken before 5.00 am, but I do not recall being tired – until my forties.

Lack of sleep is a recognized stress, and it makes losing weight very difficult. Men especially like to get heroic about sleep, priding themselves on how little sleep they get. Few of them have a six pack.

So how much sleep do we need? If you are woken by an alarm clock, then I would contend you are not getting all the sleep you need.

Today the National Sleep Foundation calculate that on average we get six hours and 40 minutes sleep on a weekday; compare to pre light bulb nights when people averaged ten hours a night. Our sleep patterns are strongly linked to what we have allowed ourselves to become accustomed to.

People who sleep less are more active, and yet they will have trouble losing weight. Women who eat less, exercise more, but sleep less gain more weight than women who sleep seven hours a night.

In 2006 The American Thoracic Society put some numbers to this theory.

People who slept five hours were 35% more likely to be overweight and 15% more likely to be obese (compared to someone who got seven hours of sleep). Those who slept six hours were 12% more likely to be overweight and 7% more likely to be obese.

Sleep deprivation interferes with the body's ability to break down carbohydrates. Lingering carbohydrates means the presence of insulin, our fat hormone.

When we sleep we inhibit cortisol. Waking up too soon will stimulate the hormone cortisol, and elevated and prolonged cortisol makes us store fat, especially around the mid section. Further, sleep deprivation will drive leptin levels down and ghrelin levels up, which will trigger cravings and overeating.

Growth hormone is released when we sleep. Growth hormone is a big player in determining how much fat and how much muscle you have. Reduced levels of HGH may reduce your muscle mass which will, in turn, increase your body fat percentage.

Sleep Deprivation can alter our body and so much more beyond that. Sleep deprivation has been used as a torture tactic and, to a lesser degree, can cause depression and moodiness. In women, sleep deprivation has been linked to an increased risk of breast cancer, endometriosis, and dysmenorrhea (painful periods).

One thought with regards to the cancer risk of poor sleep is that melatonin may be a protective hormone. Melatonin production is stimulated by the dark, and so we produce melatonin when we sleep. When the light/dark cycle is interrupted by shift work or lack of sleep women have been shown to be at higher risk of menstrual irregularities, conception problems, miscarriage and breast cancer. Melatonin had been thought merely to be the hormone that helps us sleep. But we now find it has many important functions; protection against breast cancer being one of the most vital.

Lack of sleep will make it harder to lose weight. Short sleepers tend to eat more and crave more sugar. Short sleepers retain a layer of water bloat which is especially noticeable around their mid section. If you are already sleep deprived, it would be a mistake to get up an hour earlier to get in an extra hour of exercise.

As already noted, the good news about sleep is that you can play catch up. You cannot undo a bad meal, but you can catch up on sleep. If your week gets busy, the extra hours you get on a weekend can be powerful. I do believe in going to bed early and getting up at your usual time, rather than sleeping in, which can throw you out of kilter. However, it's far more vital that you get enough sleep than how and when you get it.

POST PARTY

The party went well, drinks flowed, and the night ended the next day. Your alarm rouses you and it's back to reality. Your head aches a little, but what hurts more is what you see in the mirror. Your face and body are bloated, making sweats and a baseball hat the uniform of the day.

WATER RETENTION

Water weight is a peculiar thing. Our body is about 60% water, but when we retain water that can go up to 65%. If you weigh 150lb that could bump you up to 158lb

Water weight is heavier than fat. If you take a bucket of fat and a bucket of water the bucket of water will be heavier. As a trainer I would hear more complaints about "bloat" than I would about gaining fat, because water weight is heavy. It can feel almost suffocating, whereas fat can surprise you; you don't know it's there until one day those jeans don't fit.

There are two hormones which regulate our water balance.

ANTIDIURETIC HORMONE ADH

Antidiuretic hormone controls the amount of fluid released from the kidneys. Dehydration will trigger ADH, causing the kidneys to release less water. You know this is happening because your urine will be a strong orange color. There is less water in your urine giving it a stronger, more concentrated color. ADH, also called vasopressin, will be activated by alcohol, diuretics, sweat loss, sauna, and pain. The easiest way to avoid the bloat of ADH is to keep hydrated.

ALDOSTERONE

This is the hormone that causes more complaints than any other. It is a very fast acting hormone which hits hard. When aldosterone is present it means there can be no sodium in your urine. That is huge because water will always follow sodium. If sodium cannot leave your body because aldosterone is present, then neither will water, so you start to expand.

Aldosterone can be triggered by stress and can really mess up an important day. A lady getting ready for her wedding may be so stressed that instead of looking better on her big day, she looks a lot worse. Once the wedding is over the stress subsides, and so does the water weight. A little too late.

It can however work in your favor. Vacation weight loss is not unusual. The extra sleep and relaxation you get on vacation can take pounds off you, and just in time for you to feel more comfortable in that bikini.

The late nights and parties are definitely best suited to those in their twenties. As we get into our thirties, forties, fifties and beyond we are less equipped to deal with that kind of stress.

NEW BODY, AND NOT THE ONE I ORDERED!

MENOPAUSE & MAN OPAUSE

Men and women change shape as they age. Ladies go from a bikini to a one piece and most men should probably take note, but they tend to have less shame and stay topless even when they cannot see their own feet. The tell tale sign of middle age is the thickening of the waistline. But it is avoidable, if you understand what is going on.

Remember lipoprotein lipase (LPL), that tricky enzyme (enzymes make other things happen) that can increase the amount of fat a cell can hold. When it is active LPL will drive fat into cell storage, but when it is suppressed fat does not accumulate in that area. LPL is responsible for our body shape and fat distribution.

The hormonal changes that occur with age significantly affect LPL activity, and so alter our body shape.

As estrogen declines with age, it no longer inhibits LPL activity, so more fat can begin to be stored. The fat which estrogen once held below the belt falls away, and is redistributed around the waist.

Lipolysis (fat breakdown) is slowed, leading to the common complaint of what worked before doesn't work anymore and staying in shape becomes more of a struggle.

As LPL activity increases, more fat is being sent into storage, meaning that there is less available for energy. This triggers hunger and fatigue.

If that increase in fatigue and hunger results in eating sugary snacks then the rise in blood sugar will trigger insulin, and insulin itself up regulates LPL so even more fat can be stored.

It becomes a real challenge to keep in shape as our energy diminishes and fat becomes easier to store, and harder to burn off. Ladies that have been forced into menopause after having their ovaries removed generally experience increased appetite and weight gain. Interestingly, when women in the same situation did not allow themselves to eat more, they still gained the same weight.

Men have been studied too, and men with no testicles tended to gain weight with female like fat distribution.

As they age, more of a man's testosterone is converted into estrogen. The enzyme that converts testosterone into estrogen (aromatase) becomes more active with age. Testosterone is already decreasing so any conversion to estrogen leaves even less free testosterone. The liver is responsible for breaking down estrogen, so men can help themselves out by avoiding environmental estrogens (eat organic) and by detoxing their liver by consuming less alcohol and using milk thistle, dandelion root and eating cruciferous vegetables (broccoli, Brussels sprouts, cabbage, cauliflower, kale and collard greens). Stinging nettle and Christine Passionflower are also used as anti aromatic agents.

But ladies, it all gets a lot more complicated for us – no surprise there.

ESTROGEN (three hormones) and **PROGESTERONE** (one hormone)

- E1 (estrone)
- Made in the ovaries pre menopause and then in the adrenals. Stored in body fat and reduces during pregnancy.
- E2 (estradiol)
- Made in the ovaries and reduces during pregnancy.
- E3 (estriol)
- Made in the placenta during pregnancy and a teeny bit comes from the E1 breakdown. During pregnancy there is more E3 than E1 and E2 combined.

Progesterone is made in the ovaries and in small amounts by the adrenals. Progesterone protects during the first three months of pregnancy, until the placenta can take over. During pregnancy progesterone is then produced by the placenta.

Both estrogen and progesterone protect against heart disease by increasing the 'good' cholesterol, HDL. Women are more prone to heart issues later in life, partly due to the hormonal decline that comes with age.

WHAT A PAIR

Estrogen and Progesterone are quite the duo and, although both decline with age, progesterone usually declines more rapidly. Women don't have to wait for menopause to experience the hormonal shifts that come with age. Estrogen and progesterone may both be declining, but the sharp decline of progesterone leaves us, ironically, with estrogen dominance.

Dominance here refers to the ratio between the two hormones being altered to leave estrogen in more of a dominant role. Even though estrogen has decreased, the gap between the two hormones has widened, leaving estrogen in the even more dominant role.

This started for me at 46, but for many women, it may start a decade sooner. Still not classed as even 'perimenopause' this state of estrogen dominance can start to cause havoc and if your health is not the best I imagine the situation will be worse.

It started for me with a lot of water retention. What used to be four or five days a month was now over a week. My energy was down, and my usual good mood was a little more doom and gloom with a pinch of worry thrown in. I recall one day in particular when I was driving to work, and my thoughts were a little pessimistic. This is not me, especially first thing in the morning, my favorite time of day. Knowing what I know about hormones I ordered some bio identical progesterone cream online (I was surprised I could even do that). I tried it and almost immediately I felt better.

A blood test showed me what I had already guessed, and my doctor prescribed me a progesterone cream which made my life happier and a lot more comfortable.

I understand that many women do not want to take the hormone replacement route and I have no bias either way. Some women sail through their hormonal changes but for me it was a solution that squared with my belief system and a choice I was happy to make.

I would add is that if you are against hormonal replacement because of the nightmare stories from a few decades ago, please know that, thankfully, we are in a different place now. Bio identical hormones are not the synthetic hormones sourced from animals that were used in the 1970s.

In my nutrition business, I often see women who come to see me because of weight gain in their forties and fifties. It is a little surprising that some of these women are being prescribed only estrogen (no progesterone). Many of these women are not yet menopausal, and estrogen alone makes them even more estrogen dominant. They gain a lot of weight around their middle and are somewhat emotional.

The ratio between estrogen and progesterone is critical.

ESTROGEN

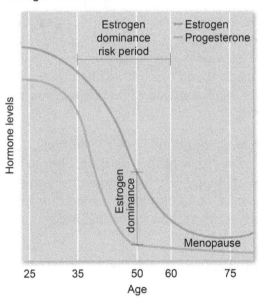

Estrogen Dominance

- Increases body fat on hips and thigh

- Increases water retention

- Increases risk of certain cancers

- Increases headaches

- Changes blood sugar

- Anxiety

PROGESTERONE

- Helps to use fat for fuel

- Natural Diuretic

- Restores libido

- Protects breast tissue

- Normalizes blood sugar

- Natural antidepressant

If you are at an age where you are experiencing estrogen dominance, certain choices will make things even worse. Estrogenic foods, environmental estrogens, an estrogen based pill or cream can all have an impact. If you are not inclined to choose bio identical hormones there is still a lot you can do to help yourself during these challenging times.

We all want to look better and have a killer body, but for me it was my depressed mood that hit me hardest. I like to be happy, and I am used to being happy. Life has thrown me some curve balls for sure, but my general state of mind is a good one, and balancing my hormones brought me back to my happy place.

TO LOOK FORWARD TO

My mum said she "sailed" through menopause in her mid fifties. I seem to recall some screaming and my dad telling me that is was just "the change" so there may be some different renditions of that time. Either way, it's useful for me to know that my mother was 56 when she indeed entered menopause. Your mother's experience may not be your own but there is a hereditary link, so it is useful information to have. My mother also tried hormone replacement back in the 1970s which may have had something to do with the screaming.

That initial introduction to hormone replacement was linked to some serious side effects, and it scared women off hormonal intervention for decades to come. As I say, thankfully times have changed, and if you're on the fence, it's certainly a conversation worth having with a doctor well versed in HRT.

Progesterone and estrogen decline until a point of "follicular depletion" (i.e. you run out of eggs).

Estrogen and Progesterone increase every month to prepare for the egg. When there are no more eggs, the cycle itself stops. Menopause is defined when a woman has missed 12 cycles; this process may take years.

The changes leading up to menopause can start to occur years earlier. Ovaries peak in a lady's mid twenties to early thirties. Generally, after 40 years of age, the number of follicles drops, and this leads to a drop in estrogen. When estrogen drops there is not enough estrogen to mature an egg and if there is no mature egg, and reduced progesterone, then periods become irregular and sometimes uncomfortably heavy.

These are the changes that get a woman's attention, but this state of flux has other repercussions. Estrogen and progesterone are useful in protecting against heart disease. They do this by keeping HDL (high density lipoproteins) high. Pre menopausal women have a much lower risk of heart disease than men their same age, but by 65 years old the rate of heart disease is almost comparable. A lady's hormones drop, so their protective function drops and the risk of heart disease increases.

Bones are continually being built up and broken down. When estrogen drops, the breakdown of bone dominates. This is a concern for women, although this bone loss does seem to stabilize a few years after menopause.

There are estrogen receptors in the bladder and the vagina. Estrogen influences collagen production which, in turn, affects connective tissue (ligaments and tendons). When estrogen drops, the pelvic floor weakens because of the changes in connective tissue. This can take a lady into an embarrassing era of UTI (urinary tract infections), incontinence and painful sex. Ladies can spend a third of their lives dealing with pre, post, and menopause itself.

Estrogen also inhibits the production of the stress hormone, cortisol. When estrogen declines cortisol levels rise, this can increase blood sugar, blood pressure and for some unfortunate women it can lead to mild to severe panic attacks. Furthermore, estrogen has a role in regulating the production of serotonin. Serotonin is a mood neurotransmitter, and estrogen helps prevent its reuptake; when estrogen declines unstable moods ensue, causing episodes of anxiety and panic.

We all know that lady who, in her younger years, could have taken on the world. She was ambitious, confident, a go getter, a life shaker, but who, in her later years, became uncertain, anxious, fragile and depressed.

The majority of women (80%) suffer to some degree with:

1. Sleep disturbances

2. Anxiety

3. Moodiness

4. Depression

5. Skin changes

6. Reduced libido

7. Hot flushes

Men don't get a pass either. Men get grumpy while women get scared; not the dream scenario for aging with your partner. Guys if your lady is becoming a little annoying, please know that are you too.

We all know that guy that in his younger years was cheerful, full of fun and curiosity but in his later years became grumpy, opinionated, argumentative and fatalistic?

It's easy to point a critical finger at the ladies, but you guys can become tough to be around. Your need to be right only intensifies as you become more emotional with the passing years. Testosterone is converted into estrogen and as men age this conversion increases. Aromatase is an enzyme that converts androgens (testosterone) to estrogens. This enzyme can be found all over the body, and it becomes more active with age, obesity, insulin and excessive alcohol intake.

MEN HAVE ESTROGEN TOO

Yes, men do have a female side, and it is not just puppies and chick flicks that bring it to the surface. Estradiol is the estrogen in men that mainly comes from the conversion of testosterone to estrogen. As men get older, the production of testosterone decreases yet the conversion of the hormones continues, especially in fatty tissue.

As men get older their male hormone drops while their estradiol levels remain high. This is due to the increased activity of that aromatase enzyme that happily converts testosterone to estrogen, and the process is enhanced by the increase of fat associated with age.

Fat releases and stores hormones, and abdominal fat produces estrogen which then enters a man's bloodstream.

How do you know if this is happening to you or your man? Their emotional disposition might be the giveaway but also feeling constantly tired, losing muscle, gaining fat on the chest and, of course, that expanding waistline.

We can become difficult as we age, putting a strain on our friends, family, and children. Some would say it is the circle of life. Your kids drive you crazy, and then you drive your kids crazy. It becomes a challenge for everyone involved and yet there are three distinct ways to help this transition into your golden years.

1. Don't get fat. As we get older we often have more time on our hands, and this can lead to mindless eating. How we look may be less important, and this also makes irresponsible food choices more likely. Controlling the hormone insulin by managing our carbohydrate intake would be a very wise choice, as insulin is the primary fat storage hormone and is associated with a host of other age related conditions, which we will shortly discuss.

2. Keep moving. Aches, pains and less energy lead to less activity, and our world becomes smaller. You used to go out a lot more. and now your world becomes your own four walls, anything beyond them is just too much of an effort. As a result of this inactivity, we have muscle loss and fat gain. The hardest thing of all in our later years might be to stay active, but we all know those older people that do; they are more energetic, more positive and more youthful.

3. Drink less alcohol. Alcohol puts a strain on the liver and the liver also has to break down fat. Alcohol seems to increase the conversion of testosterone to estrogen; it saps our energy and increases fat storage.

Chrysin (extracted from passion flower) and flaxseed are thought to help as anti aromatizing agents while zinc and stinging nettle are associated with testosterone production and the increase of free testosterone in the blood. Stinging nettle is also thought to help with the neutralization of the aromatizing agents.

Milk thistle and dandelion roots have long been used to detox the liver along with Indole 3 Carbinol, which is also found in cruciferous vegetables (broccoli, Brussels sprouts, cabbage, cauliflower, kale, bok choy, watercress, turnip, and radishes). These vegetables are rich in sulfur which helps with detoxification and may reduce the risk of breast, colon and lung cancers.

As well as the cruciferous vegetables, which seem to be a go to for every ailment of every age, women may also find relief with the following:

- **Black Cohosh**
  Hot flashes, mood disturbances, and vaginal dryness.

- **Chasteberry**
  Aka Vitex agnus cactus, used for irregular bleeding,
  PMS, increasing progesterone and so preventing some
  miscarriages.

- **Dang Guai**
  Detoxifies the blood and regulation of menstrual cycle

- **Rhodiola Rosea**
  Fatigue, poor attention, memory, and vitality.

- **Wild Yam**
  Menstrual cramps. Contains diosgenin, a plant based
  estrogen that can be converted into progesterone.

- **Ginseng**
  Vitality supports sleep and relaxation, possible
  cardiovascular support.

- **Licorice**
  Hot flashes and night sweats.

- **Red Clover**
  Potentially helpful with bone density, high blood
  pressure, high cholesterol, and inflammation.

Plant based hormones are not identical to our own hormones and can't be expected to work in exactly the same way. This concerns some health professionals. The importance and the potency of herbs can be understated, and I wouldn't advise you to just start filling your cart with these products. Female hormones are a delicate matter and deserve the attention which a naturopath or certified herbologist can provide.

Discussing the changes of age is no longer taboo. Women are the ones that usually love to talk and it is men that keep tight lipped, except when the topic is age. Women were told to age gracefully while men have been publicly tackling their declining hormones since the 1940's. The male conversation has been going on for so long that we don't even blush at an erectile dysfunction commercial on television, and no one gets judged if a blue pill helps in the bedroom. Men expect a better quality of life as they age; for decades they have demanded ways to preserve their vigor and vitality.

Ladies, please step forward.

Ladies, on the other hand, still get that critical eyebrow raise if they demand the same from their doctors. There is this martyr like strength in embracing 'the change' and rising above the superficial importance placed on youth. I, for one, am not going with that. I want to look good, I want to be energetic, I want to be positive and happy, I don't want a head full of worry and I don't want age to dictate my hair length or a one piece bathing suit.

Women deal with the rollercoaster of hormones from being a young teenager onwards, and maybe it's because hormonal change is such a big part of being a woman that it is not as acceptable to want to exert some control over the tide.

Hormonally, men have a comparatively chill ride for most of their lives. Perhaps that's why, when things do start to deviate from the mean, it's so much more unacceptable to them and to society.

"Getting old is not for the weak" a well worn phrase that sums it up quite nicely.

WHEN IT ALL COMES HOME TO ROOST

We have all heard or know of that 95 year old who is sharp as a tack and credits their longevity to their daily cigar and fast food. We also know that guy that ran 10 miles every day, ate organic and dropped down dead before he hit 50.

It's easy to sit back and place your health in the hands of fate. However, when did irresponsibility ever serve any of us well? I don't feel that this handing off of personal responsibility is an accurate reflection of a person's character. We were not taught anything about nutrition, health or disease at school, and at a young age it was probably the last thing on our mind. When our mortality catches up with us, it can be overwhelming, like trying to learn a new language which would have been much easier if we had been introduced to it when we were young. Surrounded by conflicting ideas, marketing madness, and continually emerging new information, it is understandable that people throw their hands in the air and give up. Being the prideful creatures, we are, it feels better to act like we don't care than to care but not know what to do.

But we do care. That high blood pressure result did alarm us, the number on the scale did ruin our day... We try, we try really hard and yet the scale keeps heading north, and the doctor is still frowning at our test results.

OLD

What does 'old' mean to you? At the turn of the Century it meant your forties. Today you might think mid eighties. For the more informed it might mean cellular health and telomere length. I am not putting a number on 'old.' I know plenty of old people in their thirties and I know plenty of young people in their seventies.

Being old most often refers to the time when our health takes on a definite change. So, let us use that reference point and discuss what can happen over time.

INSULIN, YET AGAIN!

In the earlier chapters, we talked about how the over release of the hormone insulin will make us fat. When we are young, that's all we cared about, not getting fat. As we get older, the toll of insulin takes on another form. Before we get to that, let's set the scene by going back. Way back...

Before birth, we feed off our mother's blood. If that pregnant lady is eating a lot of sugar and/or a very high carbohydrate diet, that shows up in her blood as blood glucose/blood sugar. High blood sugar triggers that over release of insulin from the pancreas. The baby, through its mother's blood, is also being exposed to a high level of blood sugar, so they develop more insulin secreting cells.

A baby exposed to high levels of sugar may develop the ability to produce more insulin before it takes its first breath!

Insulin is known to be the primary fat storage hormone, but insulin also acts as a growth factor. Bodybuilders have known how to manipulate this hormone to their advantage for a long time. When they want to gain muscle they 'bulk up' (an old school term which means creating a tremendous insulin response).

Insulin, protein, testosterone and growth hormone are our growth factors. The conundrum is how to build muscle and lose fat at the same time. You won't gain much muscle on a diet and, knowing this, the bodybuilder will cycle between eating to gain muscle and eating to lose fat.

That unborn baby does pretty much the same thing. Momma has a lot of sugar in her blood, and the baby makes more insulin to deal with it. Insulin works as a growth factor, and the baby gets bigger. Diabetic mothers tend to have large babies.

The baby is born, hopefully, healthy and happy and with an increased ability to produce insulin.

Before you go and chastise your mother for the state of your waistline we should recognize that just because we have the ability or the predisposition for something, it does not mean it is our destiny.

We all have the diabetic gene but what matters is if we trigger that gene. Epigenetics is a more recent conversation (although Darwin started the discussion in the 19th Century) about gene expression. To fall prey to a genetic trait, you have to pull the trigger.

If you asked my grandfather, he might have told you that high blood pressure runs in our family. Two generations later and I will tell you that bad English food runs in our family, and it is not our genetic fate.

Keeping it simple: yes, a baby exposed to a high level of blood sugar before birth may adapt in a way that works against them later in life, but only if the life they choose pulls that trigger.

Control your sugar and carbohydrate intake, keep moving every day and you won't be trigger happy later in life.

INSULIN RESISTANCE

Insulin travels in the blood and attaches to the insulin receptors on cells. When those receptors are responsive, insulin can do its job and transport nutrients into cells (muscle, fat, and liver).

Constantly eating sugar/carbohydrates means a constant release of insulin and the cells can become resistant to the persistent message of the blood clearing hormone.

A couple buys a house by a railway track. They hadn't really thought it through, and when they first move in they can't get a night's sleep because of the roar of the train every other hour. It drives them crazy. Over time they get used to the disturbance. Visitor comments on the noise; perplexed, the couple looks at each other, "What train?"

Insulin is like that train. The muscle and fat cells hear it screaming all the time because their host is making some pretty crazy food choices. Insulin keeps on screaming until eventually the muscle cells say, "What insulin?"

Insulin resistance is when the cells stop responding to insulin. Between muscle and fat, it is always the muscle cell that becomes resistant first. The muscle cell shuts down, and the fat cells have to bear the burden. and people pile on the pounds.

If we keep going past this point, the fat cells can also become resistant, and now blood sugar has nowhere to go. Neither fat nor muscle will house it, and sugar and insulin build to dangerous levels in the blood. If nutrients can no longer enter cells, the cells start to starve, and this triggers fatigue, cravings, hunger an almighty mess.

This dreadful scenario can happen at any age if you eat badly enough but, as we get older muscle does become resistant. Insulin is portrayed as the devil, but insulin is also responsible for keeping muscle intact. The presence of insulin stops muscle or fat from being broken down. As we age the muscle cells become resistant, nutrients don't get to the cell, insulin can't protect it, and muscle starts to break down. Fat cells are not resistant so as we start to lose muscle we can gain fat. When cells don't get nourished we become tired, less driven and we begin to feel OLD.

Imagine the process. We're getting older insulin resistance kicks in, with the muscle cells being affected first. Time moves on, and now the liver receptors start to become resistant. Now comes hyperinsulinism; high levels of insulin in the body, resulting in inflammation. And this feeds into a whole barrage of complaints. Next, your blood pressure goes up, triglycerides (fat in the blood) increase, HDL (high density lipoproteins the good lipid transporters) decline and it becomes more of a challenge to regulate blood sugar.

In our later years, the pancreas starts to get tired. Eating habits may have forced it to work pretty dang hard all those years. It's worn out and can't release insulin the way it once did. Blood glucose remains high, and we enter the era of type 2 diabetes.

Type 2 diabetes used to be called Adult Onset Diabetes because that's when it was expected to happen as older adults.

SIGNS OF INSULIN RESISTANCE

1. Signs of Insulin Resistance

2. Physical Fatigue

3. Mood swings

4. Mental fatigue

5. Not able to hold a thought, brain fog

6. Afternoon naps

7. Weight gain

8. Sugar cravings and overeating

9. Digestive issues, IBS, and leaky gut

10. Gas, bloating

Sounds familiar to a lot of us...

Interestingly, insulin resistance is also linked to leptin resistance. Leptin is that hormone that tells us how much we need to eat. If we become leptin resistant we're hungry all the time. This is hard to ignore, and the afflicted have a ferocious appetite.

Those afternoon naps, that forgotten thought, those bathroom issues are cast aside as the unavoidable pitfalls of getting older. But as insulin resistance takes hold, other more severe symptoms emerge.

1. Elevated Triglycerides

2. High LDL cholesterol

3. High blood pressure

4. Autoimmune disorders

5. Liver disease

6. Obesity

Don't be sucked into the belief that thin is healthy. Although weight gain is very common, insulin resistance affects the slight of body too. Indeed, those of slender frame may get harder hit just because their growing insulin resistance is less apparent.

METABOLIC SYNDROME

Metabolic Syndrome is the bringing together of a few powerhouses. Obesity, diabetes, and hypertension (high blood pressure, where the blood creates too much pressure against the walls of our arteries). All three of these conditions are associated with insulin resistance. Cancer and Alzheimer's, conditions that terrify us, are also linked to insulin resistance.

Chronic diseases are classed as those that:

- Do not get better with time.

- Have environmental triggers.

- Have multiple symptoms.

Metabolic syndrome is another step towards heart disease and one quarter of the adults in the United States have heart disease.

Coronary Heart Disease (CHD) is the main form of heart disease. Blood vessels of the heart become damaged, and this can lead to a heart attack.

There is no cure because the vessels remain damaged. Even after a bypass, which gets more blood and oxygen to the heart, you still have those buggered vessels. So how did they get buggered?

- Stress

- Processed Food

- Sugar

- Inactivity

- Obesity

- Pills, booze, and rock 'n' roll.

- Lifestyle choices that cause inflammation.

Diabetes is caused by too much blood sugar and too little exercise;

excess sugar ends up in the liver and the liver converts it into fat (triglycerides). Triglycerides travel in the blood on small dense lipoproteins (mostly VLDL). As a result, your cholesterol markers are on the up too.

Kidneys start to release sodium, and sodium holds water in the blood. This sends us right back to high blood pressure and damage to arterial walls.

For a great many years, we blamed cholesterol for all our woes. However high triglycerides are more common than high cholesterol in people with heart disease. Over half of the people with heart disease do not have high cholesterol (and we have known this since the 1960s).

High triglycerides come from too much sugar, too many carbohydrates not from cholesterol.

In 1967 there was a study of 286 patients. Out of this sample, 246 were thought to have a genetic link to heart disease. They were put on a diet with no sugar and only 500 600 calories per day coming from carbohydrates; 90% of them saw a reduction in both their triglycerides and their cholesterol.

I am not a doctor or a medical professional of any kind. My intention is merely to point out that as we have continued to learn more about disease and aging, it has become apparent that we may have got a few things backward in days gone by. Blame has zero value, and I doubt anyone meant to lead us astray, but it is also a mistake to hold on to pieces of dubious information as if they were carved in stone by Moses.

It is sufficient to say that, at this moment in time, it would be accurate to state that excess carbohydrate, and sugar dense products, coupled with inactivity and stress appear to create a central dot which joins up many other ugly dots.

Eating natural foods and doing manual labor was not a choice in the past – we just plain did it more. We scrubbed floors, walked to school, my gran washed clothes by hand, and my dad did his own garden. We ate less, cooked more, and spent more time with loved ones.

Today we have the option to eat with convenience and move only by choice. This is where we are at; discipline is only rewarded later whereas laziness is rewarded now.

What we put in our face, who we surround ourselves with and what we do with our feet has an enormous impact on how gracefully we age.

While we have been squabbling about carbs, cholesterol, and diets we enter a new era that is gaining colossal momentum. It was hard enough to give up heartfelt beliefs about calories, and now we are being asked to embrace the intangible energy we create within ourselves.

Before you slam that pre workout consider this. In 2009 I met the man who would become my husband and change my life forever. Meeting Kevin was the highlight of that year but coming in a distant second was an event that you may feel was more significant. In 2009 three people shared the ultimate prize, awarded for their work which shone new light on how we age and the power we have within ourselves to control the process.

In 2009 Elizabeth H Blackburn, Carol W Greider and Jack W Szostak won the Nobel Prize for their discovery.

'How chromosomes are protected by telomeres and the enzyme telomerase'

In short, in 2009 three people told us why we age and what we can do about it.

Despite my fascination, I have to re read this type of scientific literature many times to grasp it. I then have to get busy with a highlighter and rewrite it in my own words. The topic of telomeres is exciting and affects us all, but I do hope I don't insult the three Nobel Prize winners with my incredibly simplified summary of their life's work.

As human bodies we are made up of organs. Organs are made of tissue; tissue is comprised of cells, and each cell has a nucleus. Inside the nucleus of a cell we have chromosomes. Chromosomes contain packets of information; this information is our genetic code, our DNA.

DNA (deoxyribonucleic acid) is that spiral ladder diagram you've seen before. Each rung of the ladder is a pair of nucleotides. Nucleotides are the units that store our unique information. Chromosomes are tightly coiled strands of DNA; we have 23 chromosomes from each parent.

To say it in reverse, chromosomes are strands of DNA. Chromosomes are found in the nucleus of cells; cells make up tissue, and we have lots of tissue.

Think of a chromosome as a shoelace that has those plastic protective tips on the ends. Every piece of our data is stored in these shoelaces with plastic tips. The Nobel Prize was awarded for research on those plastic tips – our telomeres.

GROWTH AND AGE

We all started from one single cell and, for us to grow, that cell had to duplicate, and each cell after that had to duplicate (mitosis). One parent cell divides into two daughter cells, and each daughter makes copies of the information packets (chromosomes). A cell can only divide so many times (called the Hayflick limit) and when the cycle stops the cell dies. Changes in our skin and hair are annoying, but the real problem comes when the cells of the immune system can no longer divide.

Chromosomes hold all our personal data and to ensure that information is copied successfully each chromosome has that plastic tip, that telomere. With each cell division the telomeres shorten in length, and when a telomere becomes too short, the information (chromosomes) can no longer be copied, and the cell becomes old and dies (apoptosis).

It's the reduced length of the telomere that has been linked to the aging process. Telomeres protect our chromosomes, and much like that shoelace, problems arise when that plastic tip gives out.

CHRONIC STRESS

Chronic stress reduces the length of telomeres. People who care for sick children showed a reduced telomere length. The shortening corresponded to the length of care and was not a function of the caregiver's age. A young caregiver's telomere reduced in length at the same rate as a person much older. On a promising and quite miraculous note, researchers were able to stop the telomere shortening by implementing stress management techniques. In some cases, just 12 minutes of meditation a day for two months was shown to protect telomere length. For parents of hospitalized children or the long term carers of autistic kids the implications are enormous.

Ladies with cervical cancer were studied, and the results were similar. The ladies were given both mental and physical counseling, and their symptoms improved. Dr. Nelson (University of California, Irvine) went one step further and, upon reexamination, he found that the counseling had not only stopped the shrinkage, but it had also promoted telomere growth. The study participants still had cancer, that hadn't changed, but they had longer telomeres at the end of the study than they did at the start.

These incredible results tell us how positive thinking, social support, belief, attitude – faith can dramatically help with health, healing and the aging process.

THE NEW AGE OF AGE TELOMERASE

Telomere length is a function of length erosion and length addition. Stress, sickness, age will cause a telomere to shorten, and it's the enzyme Telomerase that is responsible for any growth.

Telomerase is found in fetal tissue, adult germ cells and in tumor cells. Body (somatic) tissue tends to age and die because of its very limited telomerase activity. If this enzyme (enzymes speed reactions) is activated, a cell will continue to divide. It's called the 'Immortal cell theory,' but it's not as good as it sounds. The body, as a whole is a system of regulators, brakes, and accelerators that are used

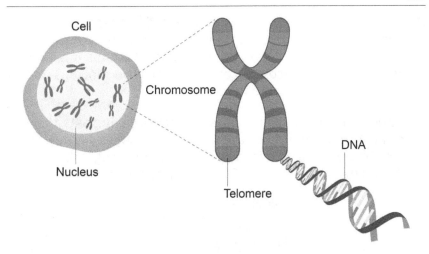

together to find a place of balance. If we slam on the accelerator, it might seem great at first, but there will be a long term price to pay. We see this with obvious behaviors, such as very restricted dieting, excessive exercise or massive sleep deprivation. You might lose weight initially, hit a personal best or get that study paper in on time – but there will be consequences.

If telomerase can keep a cell dividing it might seem great for anti aging, but quite frightening if that cell is a cancer cell.

Cancer cells are malignant cells which divide and multiply to form a tumor; telomerase is found to be 10 20 times more active in a cancer cell than in a typical cell.

An immortal body, with mere mortal disease.

What if we could activate telomerase activity in our aging body cells while turning it off in cancer cells?

The goal is not to live forever but to live forever in great health, a dream that is one step closer to being a reality thanks to the Nobel Prize Winners of 2009.

Today 40 is the new 30, and someday maybe 100 will be the new 65. We live in exciting times that are pushing us to look beyond the physical.

In times of intense stress, it can be hard to hold a positive thought.

One of those bestsellers told us how negative energy is six times stronger than positive energy. How one negative person can infect a whole office whereas one brave, positive soul cannot. It is great to know that positive outcomes come from positive thoughts, but in times of such stress it's hard to go it alone.

With a plethora of best selling books about awakening giants, thinking to grow rich and being better than good, this is not totally new to us. We pay thousands of dollars to be told how our thoughts create our reality and this is a giant size 16 step in that same direction.

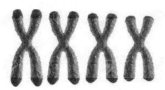

This research will expand the role of structured support for the sick and for those caring for the sick. The undeniable proof that our thoughts can change us on a cellular level brings with it a new level of personal responsibility to be kind to ourselves and to care for others. When we feel powerless there is more we can do than just hand our loved ones over to the doctors. We can listen, give of our time and be of comfort. We now know that these acts are what keeps the shoelaces tied; they are what makes another step possible.

This book was never intended to be a 'diet' book. I don't want to be one more person telling you what you should be doing. My intention is to provide you with great, distilled, comprehensible information from the frontline of health research; information you can relate to your daily life. My hope is that a new understanding will allow you to pave a path of your own design. Nutritional adjustments and lifestyle changes will move you towards your goal and while they are doing that there is one thing you can do the moment you close this book.

Belief besets attitude and attitude can literally turn back the hands of time.

Be kind to yourself.

Joanne

ABOUT THE AUTHOR – JOANNE LEE CORNISH

One of the most successful and recognizable personal trainers in the most famous gym in the world, Golds Gym Venice. Joanne has been coaching for over 25 years, her niche being getting clients stage and camera ready.

Clients over the years have included Rodney and Joan Dangerfield, Chelsea Handler, Demi Lovato, Shawn Wayans, Stephen Nichols (Soap icon), John Ridley (Oscar winner). Monica Brant (Ms Olympia) but perhaps more importantly Joanne helped Cheryl lose 100lb, got Linda strong enough to lift her own child, helped Mike feel comfortable enough to go shirtless at his beach wedding, and freed Tonya from the fear of diabetes that plagued her family. Pregnant clients, midlife clients, clients suffering from sickness, divorce, grief, injury. Joanne has worked with every issue that life has to throw at us and rarely has the answer ever been to eat less or add another hour of cardio.

A former professional bodybuilder, Joanne's experience in changing body composition spans over 30 years and three countries. Working with clients and mentoring nutrition coaches Joanne's results come from her ability to transfer otherwise confusing dull information into an edge of the seat type of experience.

Joanne and her husband Kevin live in Eagle, Idaho with a houseful of pets.

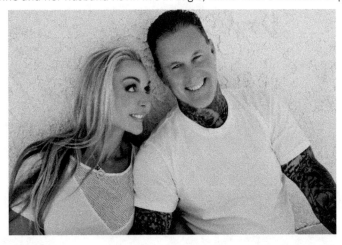

When Calories & Cardio Don't Cut It – learn how to live lean for a lifetime

More about Joanne www.joanneleecornish.com

Blog www.Theshrinkshopblog.com

Amazon www.theshrinkshopamazon.com

Workshops, Services and Products www.theshrinkshop.com

Facebook, Twitter, Instagram, YouTube The Shrink Shop

Joanneleecornish@gmail.com

Special Thanks

Illustrations E.L peopleperhour

Cover Norma M peopleperhour

PSIA information can be obtained
www.ICGtesting.com
nted in the USA
IW02n1003010918
53FS